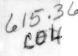

Colostrum:

Nature's Gift To The Immune System

ACTIVATE, REGULATE AND BALANCE the Immune System with Colostrum and Lactoferrin!

Revised and Updated

A Health Learning Handbook

Beth M. Ley, Ph.D.

BL Publications
Detroit Lakes, MN

BL Publications, Detroit Lakes, MN
For Orders call 1-877-BOOKS11
email: blpub@tekstar.com

Library of Congress Cataloging-in-Publication Data

Ley, Beth M., 1964-
Colostrum : nature's gift to the immune system : activate, regulate, and balance the immune system with colostrum and lactoferrin! / Beth M. Ley.-- Rev. and updated, 2nd ed.
    p. cm. -- (A health learning handbook)
Includes bibliographical references (p.68) and index.
ISBN 0-9642703-7-4
1. Colostrum--Therapeutic use. I. Title. II. Series.
RM298.C64 L49 2000
615'.36--dc21

                              00-009463

Printed in the United States of America
First edition, April 1997
Second edition, July 2000

This book is not intended as medical advice. Its purpose is solely educational. Please consult your healthcare professional for all health problems.

Credits

Cover Design: BL Publications

Art Work: BL Publications and Linda Cole

Research and Technical Assistance:
Richard H.Cockrum, D.V.M.
Raymond Lombardi, D.C., N.D., C.C.N.
Kenneth D. Johnson, S.M.D., S.N.D., O.M.D., Ph.D.,

Increasing resistance to antibiotics suggests that it is unwise to introduce one new antibiotic after another. This only leads to more and more multi-resistant strains causing infections that are increasingly difficult to control. It might be better to attempt to reinforce a natural means of resistance, which binds free iron.

C. Gillion Ward, M.D., FACS, J. J. Bullen, Ph.D., MRVCS, and Henry J. Rogers, Ph.D.,

"Iron and Infection: New Developments and their Implications," *Journal of Trauma, Injury, Infection and Critical Care* (1996)

Lactoferrin, an iron-binding protein present in milk (and colostrum) and other exocrine fluids such as saliva, bile and tears, acts as a bacteriostatic agent withholding iron from iron-requiring bacteria.

B. Lonnerdal and S. Iyer, Department of Nutrition, University of California, Davis

Technology is losing the arms race with evolution. Many scientists believe that the continued widespread use of antibiotics in medicine and agriculture makes increases in resistant microbes inevitable. In the half-century since the development of penicillin, virtually every infectious microbe has developed resistance to one or more of the major classes of antibiotics.

Bruce R. Levin, Ph.D. and M. Lipsitch, Ph.D., Department of Biology, Emory University and Department of Epidemiology, Harvard School of Public Health

"Colostrum is an important immunological liquid with proven bacteriostatic and inhibitory activity preventing the penetration of pathogenic microorganisms and absorption of potential allergens into the digestive tract."

Z. Ulcova-Gallova, Ph.D., Gynecological-Porodnicka Clinic, LF UK, Plzen.

"I use bovine Colostrum and Lactoferrin in the protocols for numerous conditions. Colostrum shows a broader base and wider application than any other natural substance. I use colostrum and lactoferrin to:

– Retard tumor growth and metastasis.

– Enhance natural "killer-cell" activity (which target specific types of tumors and virus-infected cells).

– Activate neutrophil cells (which surround and digest foreign bodies).

– Prevent bacterial overgrowth in the gut.

– Prevent viruses (including those that cause AIDS, herpes, heart disease, and some types of cancer) from penetrating into healthy cells.

– Reduce inflammation–which can reduce pain and increase mobility.

– Inhibit Candida strains.

– Inhibit free radical production-fighting the aging effects of cellular oxidation."

Kenneth D. Johnson, S.M.D., S.N.D., O.M.D., Ph.D., International
Orthomolecular Nutritionist

"Most infectious diseases enter the body through or remain local-ized on mucosal surfaces. What this means is in order to be healthy, we must be able to combat disease-causing organisms where most of them attack us, which is on the mucous mem-branes of the intestinal tract."

R.H. Weldman, Ph.D.,
West Virginia University School of Medicine and Pharmacy

"The responses have been clinically exciting in my patients using colostrum-lactoferrin lozenges for immune enhancement; especial-ly during the cold and flu season. Lozenges provide protection on the mucosal surfaces of the most where most colds and flu begin."

Raymond M. Lombardi, D.C., N.D., C.C.N.,
Redding, California

"Colostrum is a finely balanced population of proteins produced within the mammary gland. After giving birth, hormonal changes cause the accumulation and production of these finely balanced proteins to cease production. Removal before or after parturition depletes these small balanced proteins and it is replaced with an unbalanced transitional milk which compromises the quality of the colostrum.

After parturition, the mother starts to re-absorb these colostrum components. Research shows that 4 mg. of IgG is re-absorbed back into maternal circulation every hour. This greatly alters this delicately balanced material from its efficacy in regulation of immune responses.

Therefore, only excellent quality colostrum obtained in the first few hours postpartum has the highest concentration of these del-icately balanced proteins and is the most desirable for all scien-tific, animal, and human use. Only a small amount, typically a 125 mg. of excellent quality colostrum in the oral cavity, is required to activate an immune response."

Richard H. Cockrum, D.V.M., "Father of Colostrum"
Perry, Iowa

Table of Contents

INTRODUCTION

We know that long-term health is directly proportionate to the amount of time, energy and education that is spent on learning about and achieving health. Long-term, sustained health is contingent upon activating, regulating, balancing and nourishing the immune system on a daily basis. This empowers us to have encounters with deadly microbes and to survive, to engage toxins and to not get cancer, to overcome autoimmune disorders and to live a more fulfilling, healthier life.

The strength of the immune system is directly responsible for our state of health. When the integrity of our immune system is in some way compromised, it is impossible for us to obtain or maintain good health. We must be in control of our immune system.

The immune system must be stimulated without over-stiulation. Our bodies need continual regulation for proper function of the immune system. When our bodies become overwhelmed with toxins, pollutants or pathogens the regulatory features of the immune system shuts down. This often results in an immuno-compromised condition. At other times, our immune system becomes over stimulated while trying to combat various pathogens. This can result in an autoimmune disorder. Due to the large amount of these foreign substances and pathogens that we continually ingest, our immune system is constantly working. To be effective force against pathogens and toxins, the immune system requires specific nourishment.

We subject ourselves to toxins from cigarettes, drugs, highly processed foods, pesticide-laced foods, unsafe water, polluted air, antibiotics, and stress imposed by our job, family and even our friends. Under normal conditions, thanks to our immune system, these do not bother us and we do not even know they are present. An overwhelmed immune system will eventually break down, leaving us vulnerable to numerous illnesses and diseases.

As I was, you are sure to be amazed at how incredibly valuable the gift of colostrum is, not just to infants, and not just to the immuno-compromised, but to support the health of all of us!

> **"Use food as your medicine and medicine as your food."** **Hippocrates**

History of Colostrum and our Immune System

Since the beginning of time, man has observed that newborns fare better, live longer, and have fewer illnesses if they were able to obtain their mother's first milk.

In America, the Amish celebrated the beginning of a new life when a calf was born. After the calf's first feeding, they harvested the colostrum (or first milk) and prepared a pudding from it for the whole family to enjoy. The Amish noted for decades the health benefits of such a ritual. It appears that the ritual was eventually lost or replaced.

In India, where cows are sacred, colostrum is still delivered to the doorstep along with the normal milk delivery. When illness strikes a household, colostrum is often the first medication used by the family.

The way we view life and health has changed dramatically over the last hundred years. So have our lifestyles and our morality. In America, and more recently in other parts of the world, we have become a quick-fix, disposable society. Convenience and self-indulgence have become a mainstay of our lives.

As our grandparents and parents become older and die, so do many of the traditions that they passed on through generations. We have often chosen to forsake tradition for convenience and self-indulgence. As a society, are continually looking for the easy way out. This quick fix philosophy has resulted in the gradual erosion of tradition.

This philosophy has impacted every facet of our life: Our health, the stress we subject ourselves to, the way we view medicine and the pollution of our environment. Now we face Ebola, West Nile virus and other frightening diseases. These new diseases are occurring at an alarming rate. Pathogens are being observed where previously there were none–superbugs that are unaffected by our current arsenal of antibiotics. Toxins are now commonplace that were unheard of just decades ago. Obesity is at a record high, notwithstanding a myriad of low-fat and fat-free foods. Even with all the high technology the world has to offer, we have succumbed to a much poorer quality of life than that of previous generations.

Why We Die So Young

Natural human life span is believed to be at least 120 years, yet most of us die prematurely at age 73 for men and at age 77 for women. Why? If we do not provide the body with what it needs to function properly, we cannot adequately fight off illness and disease. Inadequate immune function leaves us vulnerable to recurrent or degenerative conditions or those concentrated in specific organs, such as the lungs, heart or reproductive system. Eventually, cancer, heart disease, AIDS or some other disease takes over.

Good health should not be thought of as the absence of disease. We should avoid this negative disease-orientated thinking and concentrate on what we must to do to remain healthy. Health results from supplying what is essential to the body on a daily basis, while disease results from living without what the body needs.

OUR IMMUNE SYSTEM

Without optimal immune protection we are susceptible to conditions ranging from the common cold, the flu, various stages of immune deficiency, cancer and even AIDS.

It is the responsibility of the immune system to protect us from these conditions. We may take immunity for granted until we are threatened with losing it. Research now shows that much of the efficiency of the immune system may depend greatly upon ourselves.

Immunity

Immunity is the ability of the body to overcome infection, injury and disease-producing organisms, and to recognize certain substances as foreign and to neutralize or eliminate them. The human body continually attempts to maintain homeostasis by counteracting the harmful stimuli it encounters. The immune defenses represent a variety of body reactions including the production of a specific antibody against each stimuli. It combats microbial invasion, provides resistance against the development of communicable and virulent diseases and eliminates undesirable substances from the body.

The immune system is responsible for maintaining homeostasis in every part of the body. It has duties that range from cleaning the lungs of foreign particles we inhale, to searching out and destroying invaders like infectious microorganisms and ridding the body of cancerous cells to affecting our attitudes and our sex drive. The effects of the immune system reach every aspect of our life.

The importance of the immune system cannot be overstated. The immune system is essential for human survival. It protects us not only from "invaders" such as yeast, bacteria and viruses, but also from substances such as alcohol, tobacco and caffeine. Without a properly functioning immune system, good health cannot be maintained because an individual cannot clean out or destroy the invaders.

The human body continually attempts to maintain homeostasis by counteracting the invaders it encounters. The immune defenses involve a variety of body reactions including the production of a specific antibody against the antigen it encounters. This is known as the antigen-antibody response. Whenever that specific antigen (ragweed pollen, for example) enters the body again, the immune system "remembers" and immediately forms its antibodies against it.

The normal functioning of the immune system is vital for good health and life. "***In the complete absence of the immune function, human survival is not possible for more than a day or so before overwhelming infection leads to death.***" (Snyderman)

We are confronted constantly with a multitude of various microorganisms every single day. Our ability to defend ourselves against these invaders that surround us depends on the health of our immune system. Normally our immune system is able to properly fight these off and we do not even know it is happening. Some people are not so lucky. Some people catch every cold and bacterial infection that comes their way.

In general, as we get older the immune system gradually decreases in its vitality. By age 60, the immune system may be functioning at only 20% of normal capacity, especially if any of the conditions above are present. The deficient immune system is unable to effectively fight off intruders it would otherwise fight off, such as the common cold, flu, bacteria, viruses, allergens and even cancer. The degree to which we are affected depends on a number of factors, such as our general state of health and how we respond.

How the Immune System Works

The immune system is one of the most complex systems of the body. It is highly interactive with itself and with the other systems of the body. It is impossible to remove or replace the immune system.

The immune system consists of the thymus, thyroid, spleen, bone marrow, adrenal glands, lymphatic vessels, lymph nodes (including the tonsils), specialized white blood cells such as the B-cells, T-cells (killer, helper, and suppressor), macrophage "scavenger" cells, and antibodies. Each has a different responsibility but they all function together.

There are probably a trillion white blood cells (also called lymphocytes) circulating in the body at all times, or about 3,000 of them in every drop of blood. Over 1,000,000 are created and destroyed every minute. The lymphatic and circulatory systems serve as "roadways" for the elements of the immune system to travel through the body.

Right lymphatic duct
Right subclavian vein
Submaxillary nodes
Cervical nodes
Internal jugular vein
Left subclavian vein
Axillary nodes
Thoracic duct
Intestinal nodes
Cisterna chyli
Iliac nodes
Inguinal nodes

The lymphatic system (along with the circulatory system) serves as roadways for our trillion white blood cells.

The primary objective of these cells is to recognize and attack all substances seen as foreign and to preserve those seen as self. Everything that they don't feel belongs in the body is attacked.

Any substance capable of triggering an immune response is called an antigen. An antigen can be a virus, a bacterium, a fungus, a parasite or even a portion or product of one of these organisms. Tissues or cells from another individual, except an identical twin whose cells carry identical self-markers, also act as antigens; because the immune system recognizes transplanted tissues as foreign, it rejects them. The body will even reject nourishing proteins unless they are first broken down by the digestive system into their primary, non-antigenic building blocks.

The skin is often our first line of defense as it serves as a physical barrier against bacterial, viral or chemical invasion. Body openings such as the oral and nasal cavities, gastrointestinal (GI) tract, genitourinary tract and respiratory tract are guarded against attack by the mucosa rich in lactoferrin, powerful proteolytic enzymes and secretory antibodies that can immobilize and/or destroy invading antigens. Lactoferrin is the first line of defense for any opening in the body. Often there are inadequate amounts of lactoferrin to adequately protect these areas.

Importance of the Oral Cavity

The importance of the oral cavity as part of the immune system cannot be over stressed. Most infectious micoorganisms enter the body through the oral cavity – inhale them through our nose, mouth or are ingested.

A sore throat is often the first sign of an oncoming cold. As we inhale a cold virus, it may attempt to latch onto it's new host by setting up housekeeping by replicating right there in the back of our throat. As our white blood cells identify it as foreign and alert other white blood cells to rush in to destroy the newly forming colony. We can

When visiting a doctor, the first part of the examination is to observe the oral cavity. "Say ahh."

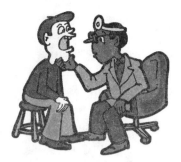

usually feel the effects of this "battle" as the sensitive tissues in the back of the throat become irritated and inflamed. If the virus is able to replicate enough it will move on - most likely into the sinus and nasal passages. If our immune system is still unsuccessful to combat it, the infection will possibly infiltrate the respiratory system, the lungs.

To prevent the virus (or any other pathogen) from going any further than it's initial place of entrance, the oral cavity is specially designed with mucus membranes and salivary glands. The salivary glands secrete several powerful important immune components including essential mucus, lactoferrin and enzymes like amylase and lysozyme. Immune cells in the mucus tissues also release secretory IgA.

The oral cavity is loaded with receptor sites which when activated, alert the entire body through a complex chain reaction of immune system events.

The Mucosal Layer Protects the GI Tract

The GI tract is normally well protected from attack by antigens in ingested food. Often the GI tract's layer of protection will break down leaving us open to pathogens. The mucosal epithelial layer is the interface between the external and internal environments in the GI tract. This is the site for the digestion and absorption of most essential nutrients. The mucosal layer also functions as a barrier that prohibits these internal bacteria from entering the rest of the body. The tissue of the intestines is defended by various resistance factors including lactoferrin, that regulates the growth of bacteria in the intestine and assists the body in maintaining its mucosal layer of protection.

The immune system alerts the body when it identifies a foreign invader by sending a signal and is also responsible for cleaning up after the invader has been conquered. Antibodies form and specialized white blood cells begin to remove the unwelcome substance.

Neutrophils, for example, rush to the site of the invasion and open up to release lactoferrin as the first line of defense. The immune system removes denatured proteins and used-up tissues from the body. If aged red blood cells were not removed each day, one could not survive for more than a few weeks because the blood stream would choke itself with all these useless particles. If just a teaspoon of the iron contained in red blood cells were available to bacteria, they would multiply and fill a large swimming pool in just 24 hours.

Specialized White Blood Cells

These hard-working defenders have a common objective to destroy all substances, living or inert, that are not naturally part of the human body. These can be derived from various sources: microscopic pollens; food allergens such as milk or wheat; other allergens such as dust or animal dander; internally produced substances, even cancerous cells; denatured proteins; and bacteria, viruses and fungi, such as Candida. If the immune system is weak, the common cold virus or ordinary pollen can become as dangerous as the sting of a scorpion.

B-Cells: These cells search out, identify and bind with specific intruders. B-cells reside in the spleen and lymph nodes and are responsible for production and secretion of antibodies.

T-Cells: These cells form killer T-cells, suppressor T-cells and helper T-cells. Such cells are specialized in killing cells of the body that have been invaded by foreign organisms, as well as cells that have become cancerous. They migrate to the invading microorganisms and destroy the them.

Killer T-Cells: These cells migrate to where antigens are present, attach and destroy the antigens.

Helper T-Cells: These cells identify enemies and rush to the spleen and lymph nodes where they stimulate the production of other cells to fight the infection. They "activate" the killer T-cells.

Suppressor T-Cells: These cells slow down or stop the activities of B-cells and other T-cells, playing a vital role in calling off an attack after an infection has been encountered.

 Macrophages: These "scavenger cells" engulf bacteria or cellular debris throughout the body by the process of phagocytosis. They also alert T-cells to the invaders' identities so they can initiate a response, and therefore play a crucial role in initiating the immune response. Macrophages are vital to the regulation of immune responses and inflammation; they churn out an amazing array of powerful chemical substances including enzymes, complement proteins, and regulatory factors such as interleukin-1. At the same time, they carry receptors for lymphokines that allow them to be "activated" into single-minded pursuit of microbes and tumor cells.

As phagocytes, which means "cell eater," macrophages rid the body of worn-out cells and other debris. They are large white cells that can engulf and digest microorganisms and other antigenic particles. Some phagocytes also have the ability to present antigens to lymphocytes.

Monocytes: Also considered phagocytes, neutrophils circulate in the blood, then migrate into tissues where they develop into macrophages ("big eaters").

Neutrophils: Neutrophils are not only phagocytes but also granulocytes: they contain granules filled with potent chemicals. These chemicals, in addition to destroying microorganisms, play a key role in acute inflammatory reactions.

Antibodies

Antibodies, also called immunoglobulins, are protein molecules commonly produced in response to the presence of an antigen. Antibodies target a specific invader. They go to the infection site where they either neutralize the enemy (antigen) or tag it for attack by other cells or chemicals. Antibodies are effective killers within the immune system. Once established, they can clone themselves whenever they are needed to fight off that particular antigen or illness again.

There are five classes of antibodies

IgG: Enhances phagocytosis to neutralize toxins (80 to 85% of total antibody serum).

IgM: Enhances phagocytosis, especially against microorganisms (5 to 10%).

IgA: Protects mucosal surfaces (about 15%).

IgD: Stimulates B-cells to produce antibodies (.2%).

IgE: Associated with allergic reactions (.002%).

We are all provided a genetically active immune system and an acquired immune response. This means part of our immunity is inherited and the rest if obtained through accumulated responses to foreign body exposures.

COLOSTRUM

Colostrum is the pre-milk fluid produced by female mammals in the mammary glands just before they give birth. While it is technically not milk at all, colostrum is often called "first milk" as it is obtained in the first milking after birth. Birth is the triggering event that ceases colostrum production in the mother and signals the body for the milk to come in or for the mammal "to freshen".

Colostrum is the fluid held in the mammary tissue until either the:

1) Newborn nurses
2) Mother reabsorbs the nutrients or
3) The colostrum is harvested

After the first milking, the fluid begins to change into milk, containing less colostrum and more milk as time passes. This transitional period lasts 2-3 days. This fluid is referred to as transitional milk.

In all other mammals other than humans, colostrum is crucial to the survival of the newborn. This is because of the high concentration of immuno factors that are transferred through the colostrum. In humans only, some immunofactors are transferred through the placenta. The colostrum is still very important, but if the newborn baby does not receive the colostrum, death is not eminent, as it is in all other mammals. (Hadorn)

> **Colostrum and lactoferrin supplements can be used on a daily basis to enhance the immune system as a preventative against illness.**

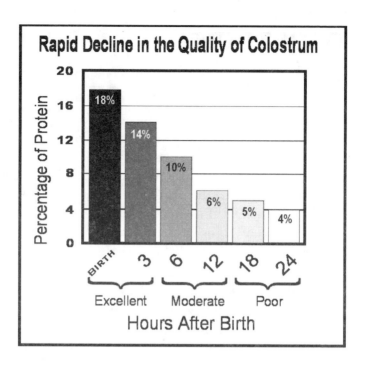

Rapid Decline in the Quality of Colostrum

TIMING is also very important. If the calf, foal, puppy, etc. experiences difficulties at birth and is unable to nurse for 12 to 18 hours, it will probably die. This is due to the re-absorption of immuno-factors by the mother. It is actually more humane and beneficial for the newborn for the colostrum to be harvested as soon as practical after birth and then bottle-fed to the newborn for the first day of life. (It is more sanitary for livestock to be bottle-fed at this sensitive stage.) This allows the newborn to receive excellent quality colostrum during the critical first 24 hours of life. Unless the colostrum is harvested immediately after birth, the quality is greatly compromised.

When selecting a colostrum supplement, it is important to keep the time of collection in mind. Also note that in virtually every scientific study performed on colostrum, the researchers diligently pursue the highest quality they can obtain at the time of the study. Research results indicate that both the quality of the colostrum and method of delivery (into the oral cavity) are very important.

Keep in mind that all of the nutritional benefits (vitamins, minerals, essential fatty acids, etc.) of breast milk and colostrum are not really applicable to supplemental forms. Breast milk is the infants only food and they may consume several pints a day. The small amount of colostrum in a supplement does not supply adequate amounts of these nutrients for an adult. The focus of colostrum as a supplement is the immunofactors, which are not required in huge amounts to stimulate and support the immune system.

Breast Milk: A Perfect Food

In humans as well as other mammals, a newborn's very first meal of colostrum is of great significance to its health and well being for the rest of its life. The immune system of the newborn is not fully developed, making it highly susceptible to numerous pathogens, antigens and allergens. Colostrum provided in breast milk contains all the needed immune factors that are essential to activate, regulate and balance the immune system. This is of great significance as the newborn's own system develops.

Mother's milk provides the perfectly assigned, individualized nutritional food to promote passive immunity and proper growth and development. As mammals grow, essential glycoproteins in breast milk keep the immune system functional.

Nutritional Support + Immunity
Mother's milk provides both immunity (passive and active) and nutritional benefits. The lipids, carbohydrates, amino acids and other nutrients provide the baby with ideal nutrition and, therefore, enhance the overall health of

the baby. Colostrum provides rich immune factors to sensitive newborns who cannot yet fend for themselves. Peyer's patches, found throughout the intestinal tract, and groups of immunoactive cells in the bronchial mucosa that destroy allergens, antigens and pathogens, are not yet operative in the newborn.

Colostrum contains antibodies against E. coli, Salmonella, Shigella. V. cholera, Bacteriodes fragilis, Streptococcus pneumonia, Bordtella pertussis, Clostridium diphtheria, Streptococcus Mutans, Clostridium tetani and Candida albicans. (Ogra)

Beast-feeding was also found to be effective against the hepatitis C virus (HCV). Research shows that both anti-HCV antibody and HCV-ribonucleic acid are present in colostrum. (Lin)

Babies deprived of breast milk are simply not as healthy as those who are breast-fed. Non-breast-fed babies develop eczema, food and upper respiratory allergies and gastrointestinal problems at a much higher rate than breast-fed babies do. (Juto)

Acquired maternal antibodies are also transferred through breast feeding and will protect the baby. For example, if the mother has contracted a disease such as measles, pertussis, or mumps, sometime prior to pregnancy, she has developed antibodies against them making her immune to reinfection. These antibodies are passed on in her breast milk to protect the baby from contracting these conditions while breast feeding. This is a most critical time of growth and development. Breast-fed babies who do contract these conditions later will experience a milder condition with far fewer complications compared to nonbreast-fed babies.

Protection from Allergies, Inflammatory and Autoimmune Diseases

Researchers hypothesize that the natural autoantibodies in colostrum and milk may contribute to the selection process of physiological development during the early postnatal period in breast-fed infants. This could explain the lower frequency of allergic, inflammatory, autoimmune diseases and lymphomas which are seen in individuals who were breast-fed as infants. (Vassilev)

Colostrum Benefits Infants with Diarrhea

Studies report colostrum helps manage infants with chronic diarrhea. In eight children with chronic diarrhea, ranging from nine months to three years of age, E. coli was present in all eight cases, Ascaris lambricoidis in four, and Giardia lambia in one. All eight children were given 20 ml. fresh human colostrum daily for seven days. In addition, those who had giardiasis received metronidazole treatment, while cases with ascariasis were given antihelminthic therapy. The results indicated that colostrum provided effective antidiarrheal action in some patents with chronic diarrhea of infective origin. (Saha)

Growth Factors

Studies show the activity of human colostrum in stimulating DNA synthesis was 20 times greater than that of bovine serum. The activity of growth factors in human colostrum was higher than that in human milk or bovine colostrum, and only human colostrum contains two different kinds of growth factors: CAGF, an epidermal growth factor, and CBGF, a platelet differentiation growth factor. (Ye)

Promotes Development of Infant GI Tract

Following birth, the infant gastrointestinal tract (esophagus, stomach and small intestine) undergoes profound growth, changes and functional maturation.

These changes are apparently related to the onset of colostrum ingestion, because starved or water-fed newborns showed little changes in the GI tract. This is due to the hormones and growth-promoting peptides, such as insulin, cortisol, epidermal growth factor (EGF) and insulin-like growth factor I (IGF-I) found at high concentrations in the maternal colostrum.

Human colostrum contains high concentrations of motilin and gastrin (hormones that stimulate the flow of gastric juices and cause bile and pancreatic enzyme release). Motilin and gastrin concentrations in human colostrum are the highest compared to human mature milk, cow colostrum and cow mature milk. The difference in motilin concentration was very significant between human milk and cow milk. (Lu)

These component in colostrum can also be used therapeutically for premature infants or newborns with immature or diseased GI tracts. (Xu)

Breast Milk Linked to Low Cholesterol

Breast-fed babies may be less likely to have elevated cholesterol levels as adults. A researcher at Baylor College of Medicine in Houston says a study of four-month-olds found differences in the way formula-fed infants produce cholesterol, which is crucial for the brain's development.

Breast milk has six times more cholesterol than formula, and formula-fed babies respond by producing their own. Despite the increased production, formula-fed babies still have 40% less cholesterol in their blood. Wong suggests that the formula-fed infants are receiving inadequate cholesterol causing them to produce it. This increased cholesterol production during infancy may have an "imprinting effect" that persists later in life, meaning that formula-fed babies may suffer from higher cholesterol levels as adults. (Butte, Wong)

LACTOFERRIN

Lactoferrin, a bioactive glycoprotein, is one of the body's own most powerful immunodefensives. While it is found in breast milk, lactoferrin is also found in small quantities in most body fluids such as saliva, tears, nasal secretions, intestinal fluids such as bile and in secondary granules of white blood cells called neutrophils. (Singleton)

It is synthesized by mucosal lining (such as in the mouth and intestinal tract) and by neutrophils, and is released by these cells in response to inflammatory stimuli. Very low physiologic serum levels of lactoferrin increase significantly upon infection. (Mann)

Receptors for lactoferrin were detected and isolated on activated T and B-cells, monocytes, intestinal brush border cells, platelets and neoplastic cells. (Adamik)

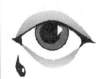 *Lactoferrin is found in tears and in other body fluids located at body openings - the oral and nasal cavities, GI tract, genitourinary tract and respiratory tract. Lactoferrin is the first line of defense for any opening in the body.*

The Benefits of Lactoferrin Include:

- Binds and transports iron in the body.

  - Beneficial for iron-deficiency anemia.

  - Provides unfavorable conditions for growth of certain harmful pathogens which need iron for proliferation.

- Promotes intestinal cell growth (enhances nutrient digestion).

- Activates and regulates the immune system.

  - Produces or stimulates production of antibodies, interleukins, killer cells and other white blood cells. (Zimecki)

  - Enhances phagocytosis, cell adherence and controls release of proinflammatory cytokines such as IL-1, IL-6 and TNF-alpha. (Zimecki)

- Provides unfavorable conditions for growth of certain harmful microorganisms (inhibits binding activity, etc.).

- Acts as an antioxidant diminishes the damaging effects of free radicals.

- Promotes maturation of immature T and B-cells.

- Controls cellular immune response and inhibits manifestations of autoimmune response in mice.

- Help speed healing of wounds.

- May have value for individuals with breast cancer.

- Potentially benefits patients with bleeding disorders as a preoperative immunomodulator. (Adamik)

Functions and Aspects of Control

Lactoferrin is closely related in structure to the plasma iron transport protein transferrin. (Singleton) The ability of lactoferrin to bind to excess iron ions, prevents the growth of bacterial and viral microorganisms and tumors, as iron is needed for their growth.

Lactoferrin also inhibits viral attack through its ability to strongly bind to the envelope protein. This prevents cell-virus fusion as the binding domain is shielded. (Swart)

Another major function of lactoferrin is its ability to stimulate the release of neutrophil-activating polypeptide interleukin 8. This suggests that lactoferrin may function as an immunomediator for activating the host defense system. Lactoferrin is implicated in particular in the control of immune functions and cell proliferation.

Researchers examining its involvement in cancer progression report that lactoferrin has a significant effect on natural killer (NK) cell cytotoxicity against certain cell lines. They also showed that lactoferrin has a normalizing effect by inhibiting cell proliferation by blocking the cell cycle progression. (Damiens)

Many other functions are attributed to lactoferrin. These include antibody synthesis, regulation and control of the production of interleukins, lymphocyte proliferation and complement activation, but the action of these functions is not fully understood.

It has been suggested that lactoferrin may contribute to T-cell proliferation. Lactoferrin regulates the iron which at low concentrations is inhibitory to T-cells. (Brock)

Lactoferrin may also have a protective function over structures such as macrophages and lymphocytes. (Brock)

Lactoferrin Regulates Inflammatory Response

One of the major benefits of lactoferrin is its ability to reduce inflammation through the regulation of inflammatory cytokines such as Interleukin-1 (IL-1, Interleukin-6 (IL-6) and tumor necrosis factor (TNF). These are a large group of chemicals largely produced by T-cells. Each one acts on a particular group of cells. While they are necessary in certain situations, too much of even a good thing can be damaging.

The problem is that high levels of these substances are seen in individuals with inflammatory autoimmune conditions such as rheumatoid arthritis, lupus, asthma, allergies, etc. Overproduction of IL-6 may explain many of the symptoms of these conditions. (Matsuda, Di Poi, Nawata, Jones) Specifically, in individuals with rheumatoid arthritis, IL-6 is produced by the synovial fluids and contributes to inflammation, tissue damage and pain. (Matsuda)

One study investigated whether lactoferrin can improve the immune competence of cells from patients with systemic inflammatory response syndrome. Three groups of volunteers (7 persons per group) took one capsule containing 2, 10 or 50 mg. of bovine lactoferrin for seven days. A control group took a placebo only.

The researchers concluded that lactoferrin was effective in helping to regulate actions on the altered reactivity of peripheral blood mononuclear cells. Specifically, they found that lactoferrin is a good inducer of IL-6 and TNF-alpha production. (Adamik)

Supplemental Lactoferrin

In most colostrum dietary supplements, the lactoferrin content is not sufficient unless additional amounts are added. Please note that a newborn calf will ingest a half-liter or more of colostrum at its first meal and will therefore receive an adequate amount of lactoferrin. Most colostrum supplements, even at high doses of up to 2 grams per day, contain less than 2% of the lactoferrin that a newborn receives. It is far better to take the highest quality colostrum obtainable and to be sure that it is supplemented with additional lactoferrin to receive the correct balance.

Lactoferrin works on contact and is therefore best utilized if taken into the oral cavity (mouth) so it can begin working right away.

COLOSTRUM-LACTOFERRIN SUPPLEMENTS

Fortunately, the numerous immune factors found in colostrum and lactoferrin are transferrable from one species to another. This means that humans can benefit from the immune-rich colostrum and lactoferrin from cows.

Colostrum from cows is much richer in immune factors than that of humans. (Sandholm) Human colostrum contains only 2% IgG (the body's most important immunoglobulin) while bovine colostrum contains 86% IgG. (Bunce)

A variety of colostrum-lactoferrin supplements derived from bovine colostrum are now available for use by adults and children. These can be found in the form of powder, capsules, tablets, chewables, lozenges, liquids, creams and etc.

Infants and Children

Ideally, women should breast-feed as long as possible. But some women are unable to breast-feed their newborn or cannot breast feed for the entire first year due to mastitis or other reasons. The benefits of colostrum can still be obtained through colostrum supplementation. By supplementing your bottle-fed child with an excellent quality, pure, unadulterated, liquid bovine colostrum, it is still possible to obtain many of the immuno and growth factors so important for proper development.

If the following regime is adhered to each time your

infant drinks, you will help to ensure proper immunity, brain and gastrointestinal development for your infant. This is an excellent way to supplement the diet for infants that are unable to breast-feed.

Please note that the following is only applicable for excellent quality bovine colostrum liquid. Suggested use for any other quality colostrum cannot be predicted nor can the results.

Colostrum Liquid Infant Supplementation

Birth to 6 Months: Add 1 drop/day in formula, water or juice. If the infant is in any type of distress, add 1 drop/feeding until distress is gone and then continue 1 drop/day.

6 Months to 1 Year: Add 2 drops/day in formula, water or juice. If the infant is in any type of distress, add 2 drops/feeding until distress is gone and then continue 2 drops/day.

Over 1 Year: Add 3 drops/day for each year of age. If in distress, use 3 drops/feeding for each year of age.

After age two, or when the child is old enough, you can start them on a regime of lozenges to continue the process. Excellent quality lozenges are available through most fine health food stores. If you can find a product that combines both colostrum and lactoferrin in an oral delivery it will save time and effort while providing the best for your child.

A maintenacne dose of one lozenge daily should provide adequate protection. At first sign of illness, you may safely increase the intake to 2 to 4 lozenges daily. The liquid may also safely be utilized.

Adults

All mammals build immunity during their lifetime based upon the pathogens they come in contact with. If a mammal grows up in a sheltered environment free of toxins and pathogens, its immunity will be much lower (weaker) than a mammal growing up in close proximity to other mammals and therefore numerous pathogens. You may recall how remote tribes all over the world were all but eliminated when explorers came into their camps and accidentally introduced a common form of influenza. Since the tribes had never encountered the flu, they had no immunity to fight it off.

Back to Basics

For years bovine colostrum was used as a folk remedy in Scandinavian countries. This changed in the 1950's when all the "highly sophisticated, medically-advanced" miracle drugs came into the picture. One could experience instant relief from infectious disease. "Just take a pill and you're cured!" (Not really, but that is what we thought.)

People chose to ignore older, traditional methods that clearly worked, but for which there was not always clear scientific data supporting them. Colostrum contains many complicated factors which work together. It does not have just one easy-to-describe mode of action, like penicillin.

Our current medical environment

The prevalence of AIDS, immune disorders such as Lyme disease, Epstein-Barr (chronic infectious mononucleosis, sometimes called Chronic Fatigue Syndrome), Fibromyalgia, Candida-Related-Complex, Herpes Simplex and various autoimmune disorders have forced us to learn more about our immune system, our health in general and the effect of negative lifestyles. These immune disorders have caused us to review all the nutritional options. One of these is the use of supplemental colostrum and lactoferrin.

Colostrum was specially designed by nature to:
- *Protect*
- *Activate*
- *Regulate*
- *Support our immune system*

Protection

Immunoglobulins

Colostrum contains all four of the key immunoglobulins: IgM, IgG, IgA and secretory IgA. These immunoglobulins are equipped with special adaptive sites which are effective at neutralizing a wide range of bacteria, viruses and yeasts. (Brandtzaeg) They include antibodies specific to fight disease-causing microorganisms.

Colostrum provides specific antibody reactivity to bacteria, viruses and yeasts. (Ogra) Most infectious diseases enter the body through the mouth or remain localized in mucosal surfaces, primarily the stomach and intestinal tract. (Weldham) We must be able to combat diseases-causing organisms where they attack us.

Fortunately, colostrum helps us do that. Most of the colostrum antibodies are believed not to be absorbed and digested but to remain in the intestinal tract after being swallowed where they fight off intruders. (Tyrell)

It is commonly assumed that the digestive enzymes in

the stomach and intestines would break up or digest the immunoglobulin-protein molecules in colostrum when ingested; Research has shown, however, that colostrum contains a powerful trypsin inhibitor and a number of protease inhibitors that protect the immune factors from breaking up. (Von Fellenberg)

The major benefits of immune factors in colostrum and lactoferrin occur within the mouth, stomach and on the intestinal and bronchial walls, and not as a result of their passage into the tissues. (Tyrell) This means if the majority of immune-enhancing benefits occurs in these locations, colostrum can benefit people of all ages. Added support can make a tremendous difference where the immune system is marginal or below marginal.

Leukocytes (White Blood Cells)

Colostrum contains living white blood cells which protect us from a variety of pathogens. Neutrophils and macrophages are the most prominent cells in colostrum. Lymphocytes are also present, predominantly T-cells, which produce interferon and other protective factors.

Safe Viral and Bacterial Protection

Dozens of scientific papers suggest that colostrum can block or reduce the severity of a wide variety of infections including many which have their initiation in the oral/fecal route.

Colostrum is effective against a number of microorganisms including the following bacteria: E. coli (including 0157 strain), Streptococcus pneumococci, Clostridium difficile toxins A and B, Vibrio cholera, Salmonella, Shigella, Bactericide fragilis, Bordtel Ia pertussis, and the following viruses: Rotavirus, Respiratory Syncytial Virus (RSV), Coxsackie, Echo and Alphaviruses, Poliomyelitis, Enteric, Hemagglutinating Encephalitis, Herpes Simplex and yeasts such as Candida.

Escherichia coli

E. coli is a species of bacteria which normally lives in the intestines of humans, and also in the feces of cattle. It is common in water, milk and soil. It is the most frequent cause of urinary tract infections and a cause of serious infection in wounds. E. coli is also responsible for diarrhea, and for the production of toxins that create intestinal irritation because of their ability to adhere to the intestinal wall.

Numerous researchers have demonstrated that colostrum has bacteriostatic and bacteriocidal effects against E. coli. Peroxidase, lactoferrin and IgA, all found in colostrum, are capable of creating powerful effects against E. coli.

Streptococcus pneumonococci

Streptococcus pneumonococci is the cause of 90% of the cases of bacterial pneumonia in the United States. Oligosaccharides found in colostrum have been shown to block attachment of a wide variety of bacteria, especially S. pneumonococci, to mucous membranes, thereby aiding in the prevention of respiratory inflammations. (Hanson)

Clostridium difficile toxins A and B

Clostridium bacteria are spore-forming and need no oxygen to live. The proliferation of this bacteria is believed to be predominantly the result of two toxins. Studies have shown that colostrum is effective in neutralizing these two Clostridium difficile toxins. (Kim)

Salmonella

Salmonella infection is commonly caused by eating contaminated food. Salmonella infection in humans can cause gastroenteritis (commonly marked by sharp pain in the stomach or intestines, watery diarrhea, nausea and vomiting), and enteric and typhoid fever. Colostrum is effective against Salmonella.

Rotavirus

Rotavirus is probably the most common cause of infant death in developing countries. Studies have shown that colostrum has protective properties against Rotavirus diarrhea outbreak.

Rota hyper-immune colostrum has demonstrated to effectively prevent the outbreak of diarrhea, however, it did not prevent immunological responses to natural rotavirus infection. In the trial, Rota hyper-immune colostrum had no effect on duration of diarrhea, bowel movements or virus shedding in stool. There were no side effects of Rota hyper-immune colostrum administration (Ebina)

Respiratory Syncytial Virus

This virus is often the cause of bronchitis and pneumonia in humans. In 1982, research at the State University of New York at Buffalo demonstrated that humans and animals exposed to Respiratory Syncytial Virus (RSV) developed protective antibodies against this virus in the IgG and IgA classes. These protective antibodies were found in large quantities in colostrum, particularly those of the IgG class. (Theodore)

Herpes Simplex Virus

Herpes simplex, which is highly contagious, is known to cause cold sores. Since the 1970's we have known that bovine colostrum are able to destroy Herpes simplex virus-infected cells. (Kohl) I could not locate any specific human studies on the effect of colostrum or lactoferrin supplementation on cold sores, but I suspect that they would decrease one's risk of outbreak as one's immunity would be strengthened.

Candida Albicans

Several studies have revealed that colostrum leukocytes proved to be effective in controlling the yeast infection Candida albicans. (Ho, Goldman)

Researchers in Denmark reported that colostrum tablets proved to be effective treatment for oral Candida among HIV-infected individuals, given ten times a day for ten days. (Christensen)

Bowel irregularity and inconsistency often accompany intestinal bacterial upset. Colostrum powder in capsule form promotes the growth of bifida bacteria and other healthy flora in the intestinal tract. These beneficial bacteria help maintain a homeostatic environment and help stimulate the musculature of the colon. A healthy intestinal microbial flora population also promotes an improved and comfortable digestive tract and helps one avoid gas and bloating.

Colostrum promotes a healthy intestinal microflora population, enhances utilization of the nutrients in the foods we eat, and provides protection against enteric pathogens. Therefore, it helps provides a stable, stronger defense against infection by pathogenic organisms, which especially seek a weakened host.

Activation

The oral cavity is loaded with receptor sites which when activated, alert the entire body through a complex chain reaction of immune system events.

Supplementing colostrum of excellent quality from the first milking in the mucosal membranes of the mouth triggers the chain reaction to occur throughout the body. This excellent quality colostrum can trigger a response that will reach all aspects of the immune system while colostrum which contains milkings past the first milking may be less effective.

In the first milking after the cow gives birth contains 2 to 2 1/2 gallons which is 100% colostrum (of which approximately 1/2 gallon goes to the newborn calf). The second milking contains only about 20% colostrum. The rest is considered transitional milk. If this, or any other milking is mixed into the first milking, the delicate balance of colostrum components is destroyed.

Remember that researchers only use first milk colostrum of excellent quality in their trials so that if we expect to get the same beneficial results, we also need to use only first milk colostrum. Only a small amount of excellent quality colostrum is needed to activate an immune response.

Regulation

Accessory factors

Colostrum also contains immuno-regulatory factors that enhance immune reaction when it is too low and suppress it when it is too high. Colostrum therefore could be a significant tool in assisting the body in regulating the immune system. This is important for conditions in which the immune system is extremely depressed, as in severe bacterial, viral and yeast infections and in cases where the immune response is generally excessive involving inflammation and destruction (autoimmune conditions such as rheumatoid arthritis, lupus, M.S. and allergies).

Lactoferrin

Lactoferrin is the premier immuno-regulator. Lactoferrin has powerful regulating effects on the production of inflammatory cytokines. An overproduction of cytokines is commonly seen in many auto-immune conditions such as allergies, asthma, arthritis, lupus and inflammatory bowel disease. Recent research suggests that lactoferrin may be very helpful to regulate this overproduction. (Zimecki)

Lactoferrin is an iron-binding protein. Individuals with

an adequate intake of iron may not be able to use the iron effectively because they may not have high enough levels of iron-binding protein to facilitate iron transport. Iron-deficient individuals experience weakness, headaches, tingling sensations in the hands and feet, brittle nails and lowered resistance to stress and disease.

Lactoferrin allows individuals to better use the iron that is in the foods they eat or in their supplements. In addition, colostrum provides essential amino acids and other nutrients in a highly desirable form. It is an excellent food source for older individuals who have compromised digestive tracts.

Proline-Rich-Polypeptides

Colostrum contains a special Proline-Rich-Polypeptide (PRP) that serves as a powerful regulator of the immune system. PRP in colostrum increases the permeability of the skin vessels, which offers a regulatory activity, stimulating or suppressing the immune response. (Staroscik)

The ability to stimulate or suppress the immune response is highly significant. Suppressing the immune system is necessary to prevent the immune system from attacking the body itself, as in the case of autoimmune diseases such as rheumatoid arthritis, lupus, M.S., Alzheimer's disease and allergies. Colostrum's suppressive action may help prevent this type of activity involved in autoimmune diseases.

This component of colostrum supplementation may turn out to be even more important than we now realize. We are only in the beginning stages of realizing the total potential of PRP and other colostrum accessory factors in for the management of autoimmune/inflammatory conditions.

Support

Transforming Growth Factors

Transforming Growth Factors (TGF) are polypeptides which promote cell proliferation, tissue repair and maintenance (wound healing) and embryonic development. Dr. F.J. Ballard, et al, found bovine colostrum contained up to 100 times the mitogenic potency of human colostrum. Studies have also demonstrated the anti-cancer ability of TGF in bovine colostrum in humans. (Tokuyama)

This aspect of colostrum also makes it especially appealing for topical use. Conditions such as eczema, dermatitis, acne, possibly psoriasis and many other other skin conditions could benefit.

Nucleotides

Nucleotides are important in cellular metabolism. The most important nucleotide in colostrum is AMP (Adenosine Monophosphate). AMP is a precursor for ADP, adenosine diphosphate, which is involved in cellular energy transfer. AMP plays a regular role in cellular metabolism and also mediates the traffic of hormones and other activators. Additional nucleotides in colostrum help metabolize carbohydrates.

Enhanced Nutrient Absorption

The elderly are at higher risk for illness and disease for a number of reasons. One is the obstacle of diminished nutrient absorption and nutrient deficiencies, which further weakens immunity. Enzymes found in colostrum help the entire digestive process to aid in nutrient absorption and utilization.

Who Can Benefit From Supplementing Colostrum and Lactoferrin?

Colostrum-lactoferrin supplementation is not just for individuals with severely compromised immunity or infants who cannot receive adequate amounts from their mother, almost everyone can benefit. Any individual wanting to feel his or her best by strengthening their immune system to ward off disease and illness can utilize a daily maintenance dosage of colostrum. As we get older our immune system begins to show signs of weakening, so this becomes even more important.

At first sign of illness, one can increase the dosage to halt or weaken the infection. Many people report results similiar to the following:

"I came down with the worst cold I can remember having in many years. I began taking the colostrum the day I felt myself getting sick. For one day I was flat on my back and the next day I woke with just minor sniffles. Normally when I've come down with a cold like that it would take at least a week or longer to get over it. I took 8 colostrum lozenges throughout that first day. From now on I will take them on a regular basis. I'm thoroughly impressed. Thank you!" (J.G.)

Colostrum For Lactose Intolerant Individuals

Lactose-intolerant individuals (regardless of body weight) can usually tolerate up to about 77 mg. lactose before a response is likely to occur. Poor quality colostrum contains higher levels of lactose compared to high quality colostrum. The sooner the collection after birth, the lower the level of lactose. The level of lactose in colostrum doubles in just 24 hours.

Unfortunately only a few companies report the level of lactose contained in their product. The following information will allow you to determine acceptable lactose levels for lactose-intolerant individuals. (Fleener)

The amount of colostrum that can safely be ingested without triggering a lactose intolerance response that is based upon the quality of colostrum:

EXCELLENT	**MODERATE**	**POOR**
700 mg.	500 mg.	350 mg.

Note: This is not the recommended dosage of colostrum. The above amounts are merely the maximum amounts that can safely be taken by lactose-intolerant individuals at one time. Extremely good results for a variety of ailments can be achieved with as little as 125 mg. of excellent quality colostrum delivered in the oral cavity.

Composition of Colostrum Supplements

The composition of supplemental colostrum differs widely from one provider to another. The following information may be useful to see how extremely important excellent quality colostrum is (quality in reference to time of collection).

QUALITY OF COLOSTRUM:	EXCELLENT	MODERATE	POOR
Total Protein:	50-60%	40-50%	<40%
Total Immunoglobulins % of Protein:	30-50%	20-30%	as a <20%
Total Fat:	13-18%	10-12%	<10%
Total Lactose:	6-11%	12-20%	>20%

Also found in trace quantities:

Vitamin A	Vitamin E	Choline
Peroxidase	Vitamin C	Vitamin D
Folic Acid	Carotinoids	Orotic Acid
Catalase	Vitamins B1, B2, B6, B12	

COLOSTRUM-LACTOFERRIN APPLICATIONS & RESEARCH

It is very difficult to form a complete list of all of the potential benefits of supplementing colostrum and lacto-ferrin. Here is a brief overview:

1. General immune enhancement - especially for immuno-compromised individuals (ill, elderly, high stress, undernourished, etc.) Helps boost resistance against illness of all kinds.

Does this mean that one will not ever get sick if using colostrum and lactoferrin? No, it does not. Most people report greatly enhanced immunity. For example, an individual who otherwise experienced 2-3 colds or flu per year after supplementing colostrum and lactoferrin may only experience 1 cold or flu per year. And, very importantly, recovery periods reduced from 5-7 days (without colostrum and lactoferrin), to 1-3 days when supplementing colostrum and lactoferrin.

2. Antiviral/antibacterial protection–specific and non-specific

3. Protects against numerous auto-immune conditions: Arthritis, allergies, asthma, multiple sclerosis, lupus, diabetes, etc.

4. Regulation of inflammatory response: Down regulates IL-6 and TNF inflammatory responses often seen in auto immune conditions and boosts white blood cell activity to increase resistance.

AIDS/HIV

A number of research groups have shown that colostrum and lactoferrin have inhibatory effects against HIV. (Swart) Lactoferrin either reduces viral absorption or penetration or both. (Harmsen)

Researchers in Rome at the Laboratory of Immunology, Istituto Superioredi Sanita, reported that bovine lactoferrin had potent antiviral activity against HIV. They found that both HIV-1 replication and syncytium formation were efficiently inhibited, in a dose-dependent manner by lactoferrins. Bovine lactoferrin markedly inhibited HIV-1 replication when added prior to HIV infection or during the virus adsorption step, thus suggesting a mechanism of action on the HIV binding to or entry into C8166 cells (a type of T-cell typically attacked by HIV). (Puddu)

Levels of plasma lactoferrin are decreased in HIV-infected patients in relation to the progression of the disease. Ninety-seven subjects were studied (22 asymptomatic and 45 symptomatic patients compared to 30 healthy controls). The results showed a highly significant decrease in the level of lactoferrin in HIV-infected patients compared to controls.

Immunoglobulins from bovine colostrum contain high levels of antibodies against a wide range of bacterial, viral and protozoal pathogens as well as against various bacterial toxins. It is quite resistant to 24-hour incubation with gastric juice (they are not broken down in the stomach and therefore able to provide a variety of protective benefits).

Colostrum for Candida/Mouth Sores

Oral candidiasis is common among HIV positive individuals. Lactoferrin, lysozyme, secretory IgA and numerous other important protective factors in a colostrum lozenge can offer excellent localized (and systemic) immune protective benefits to individuals with compromised mucosal immunity.

In the late 1980's, researchers from Denmark reported at the European Conference on Clinical Aspects of HIV Infection in Brussels that colostrum tablets proved to be effective treatment for thrush (oral candida) among HIV-infected individuals, given ten times a day for ten days. (Christensen)

Colostrum, as a natural antibiotic, is also effective for painful ulcers in the mouth. A colostrum lozenge (containing 60 mg. immunoglobulins),10 times a day for seven days encouraged spontaneous healing in a placebo-controlled study. Healing time was shortened and pain was diminished even in the first day in some patients. (Lassus)

Colostrum Stops Diarrhea Caused by C. Parvum

Cryptosporidium Parvum (C. parvum) is an opportunistic parasite infection common among individuals with HIV. It is the most common cause of the frequently experienced diarrhea. Diarrhea and weight loss are found in more than 50% of patients with AIDS.

In a multi-center pilot study, 37 immunodeficient patients with chronic diarrhea were treated with oral bovine colostrum immunoglobulins (10 g./day for 10 days). Good therapeutic effects were observed. Out of 31 treatment periods in 29 HIV-infected patients, 21 gave good results leading to transient (10 days) or long-lasting (more than four weeks) normalization of the stool frequency. (Rump)

A number of additional clinical studies have also shown that colostrum is very beneficial in treating individuals infected with C. parvum diarrhea. Supplementing dried colostrum promoted weight gain and restored energy. (Nord, Plettenberg)

Allergies and Asthma

Research shows that individuals with hayfever (allergic rhinitis) and asthma have higher levels of inflammatory cytokines (IL-6 and TNF-alpha) compared to controls. (Saito, Subratty) Lactoferrin helps regulate and reduce these inflammatory factors, which can reduce the onset and severity of problems.

Inflammation can also become more manageable with the regulating factors (such as PRP) in colostrum, which lowers one's sensitivity point, suppressing the immune reaction. Lactoferrin helps reduce inflammatory factors which can reduce the severity of reactions. The self-reacting autoantibodies in colostrum serum play a major role in the selection of the pre-immune B-cell repertoire and in the maintenance of the immune homeostasis.

The PRP in colostrum helps regulate or lower the sensitivity point of the lungs, suppressing the immune action. Colostrum forces the differentiation of certain cells so that the lungs are less sensitive. The initial reaction may still occur, but far less severely, making the asthma much more manageable.

Lactoferrin may play a regulatory role as it inhibits tryptase activity. (Cregar) The physiological function of neutrophil lactoferrin may be the inhibition of tryptase released from mast cells tryptase involvement in both late-phase bronchoconstriction and airway hyperreactivity. (Elrod)

One interesting study examined the effects of lactoferrin in allergic sheep on asthma. The study showed that lactoferrin inhibits tryptase, a potential causative agent of bronchial spasm that is released by activated mast cells (such as by an antigen or irritant). (Cregar) Aerosolized lactoferrin (10 mg. in 3 ml. buffered saline solution) was given 1/2 hour prior to as well as 4 and 24 hours after they were exposed to an inhalation challenge. The lactoferrin diminished the bronchial constriction and airway hyperresponsiveness 4 and 24 hours after exposure to an antigen. (Elrod)

It would be interesting to see additional studies on humans to see what benefits of supplemental lactoferrin are available to asthmatics.

Cancer

Japanese researchers showed that transforming growth factor-beta-like peptides in bovine colostrum inhibited the growth of cancer cells. The investigation showed that TGF-beta-like peptide purified from bovine colostrum, remarkably suppressed growth of cancer cells. The researchers also noted an intriguingly striking change in cancer size. (Tokuyama)

Other researchers have also found that colostrum has a inhibitory effect on certain cancers associated with immune deficiency). The inhibitory activity was not toxic, and was free of side effects. (Hooton)

A Finnish study demonstrated that a medium based on bovine colostrum and adult bovine serum can be used successfully as a fetal bovine serum substitute in the culture of several anchorage-dependent and independent cell lines, including a type of bone cancer and mouse mammary tumor cell line. (Viander)

Lactoferrin Possesses Anti-tumor Effects: Lactoferrin also reduces the damaging effects of free radicals, known cancer risk factors. Lactoferrin promotes other immune activities in the body by promoting maturation of immature T- and B-cells. One molecular form of lactoferrin with a ribonuclease activity may have value against breast cancer. (Adamik)

Researchers examining its involvement in cancer progression report that lactoferrin has a significant effect on enhancing natural killer (NK) cell ability to attack haematopoietic and breast epithelial cell lines. The study also demonstrated that lactoferrin inhibits epithelial cell proliferation by blocking the cell cycle progression. (Damiens)

Researchers have demonstrated that lactoferrin inhibited tumor growth in mice of transplantable solid tumors. Lactoferrin also substantially reduced lung colonization by melanoma cells in mice. Iron-saturated and apo-lactoferrin exhibited comparable levels of tumor inhibition and antimetastatic activity. The researchers claimed the results for lactoferrin suggest a potentially important role for this molecule in the primary defense against tumor growth and formation. (Bezault)

Since 1985 cytokines found in colostrum (interleukins 1-6 and 10, interferon G, and lymphokines) have been one of the most researched protocols in scientific research for the cure of cancer. Also, colostrum lactalbumin has been found to be able to create the selective death (apoptosis) of cancer cells, leaving the surrounding noncancerous tissues unaffected.

The mixture of immune and growth factors in colostrum can inhibit the spread of cancer cells. If viruses are involved in either the intiation or the spread of cancer, colostrum could prove to be one of the best ways to prevent and control the disease.

For all of the above factors, I strongly recommend cancer patients to include colostrum in their fight against cancer.

In addition, for cancer chemotherapy patients, colostrum lessens adverse effects of cytotoxic agents. It actually enhances chemotherapy so people can take greater dosages without getting so deathly sick.

Kenneth D. Johnson, S.M.D., S.N.D., O.M.D., Ph.D., International Orthomolecular Nutritionist

Much more work needs to be done in this area to determine the full cancer-protective potential of colostrum and lactoferrin.

Chronic Fatigue Syndrome

Chronic Fatigue Syndrome (CFS) is believed to be caused by the Epstein-Barr Virus (EBV), the same virus that causes mononucleosis. EBV is a member of the herpes family and is related to the viruses that cause genital herpes and shingles. The virus causes an over-reaction of the immune system. The immune system becomes so overburdened the result is immunity "burnout." The result is a feeling of complete exhaustion.

Individuals with EBV require a comprehensive restorative program for the immune system. And what is better than colostrum and lactoferrin to activate, regulate and balance the immune system?

A number of studies show that colostrum and lactoferrin inhibit the replication of several strains of herpes viruses, including Herpes Simplex type 1 and 2 (Marchetti, Siciliano, Hasegawa). Lactoferrin is also known to prevent virus absorption and/or penetration into host cells, indicating an effect on the early events of virus infection. The researchers state that lactoferrin possesses a potent antiviral activity and may be useful in preventing certain herpes viral infection in humans. (Hasegawa)

In my experience, the patients who gain the most from colostrum-lactoferrin are those with compromised immunity, chronic and recurrent disease symptoms such as chronic fatigue syndrome, Crohn's disease, infectious diarrhea, sinusitis, and fibromyalgia.

Kenneth D. Johnson, S.M.D., S.N.D., O.M.D., Ph.D., International Orthomolecular Nutritionist

Depressed levels of IGF-1 increases cellular and tissue sensitivity. Low IGF-1 levels are associated with many of the complications of diabetes, especially in Type II diabetes (Cortizo), such as kidney problems (Segev), weight gain and obesity (Bereket), diabetic retinopathy (Lacka), injury and delayed wound healing (Brown) and possibly vascular complications and cardiovascular disease (Goke, Bereket).

Iddition of IGF-I treatment to insulin in adolescents with IDDM can restore circulating IGF-I levels and thus suppress GH levels and improve insulin sensitivity and glycemic control and decreases insulin requirements. (Dunger)

Several studies show that bovine colostrum supplementation increases serum IGF-1. (Mero, Wester)

Dr. Raymond Lombardi reports that the diabetic patients in his Alternative Health Care Practice in Redding, California, who are taking 3-6 colostrum-lactoferrin lozenges daily all report fasting glucose reading an average of 10 points lower, and a reduced frequency in infection.

Other diabetic individuals using colostrum-lactoferrin ozenges report the following:

- Within 3 days, fasting blood sugar levels upon awaking are normal.

- Within 7 days, insulin use is reduced to 1/2.

- Within 30 days, their fingernails have hardened.

rrhea

Colostrum and lactoferrin are helpful st the major causes of diarrhea:

acteria: E. coli is a bacteria that lly lives in the intestines of people nimals and elsewhere. Most strains coli are quite harmless. E. coli 7 is an exception, as a major

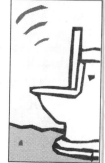

Studies also indicate that individuals with acute viral infections have reduced lactoferrin content as compared with normal. This suggests an acquired defect of neutrophil lactoferrin synthesis in viral infection. (Baynes)

Hopefully, there will soon be human clinical trials to demonstrate the effect of colostrum and lactoferrin on EBV. Meanwhile, people with Chronic Fatigue Syndrome continue to report the good results they have been experiencing.

Colds, Flu and Sore Throat

In a controlled study to determine the effectiveness of colostrum on a sore throat (often one of the first signs of an oncoming cold or flu) individuals showed significant reduction of some symptoms from the first day. (Aabakken) Other related studies (against tonsillitis forming bacteria) have shown similar beneficial results. (Urban)

Individuals report both the severity and the duration of symptoms of colds and flu are significantly reduced when using colostrum supplementation.

Dental Problems

Our saliva was carefully designed to protect our teeth and gums. It contains many antimicrobial agents (including lactoferrin) known to have anti-bacterial effects on cavity-causing bacteria.

Studies by researchers in Finland have shown that enhancing these properties of saliva can be done by adding antimicrobial proteins such as peroxidase, lactoferrin and lysozyme to oral health products. The researchers stated that although clinical evidence is still limited, using such "natural antibiotics" rather than synthetic agents against cavity-causing bacteria seems promising. (Tenovuo)

Colostrum and lactoferrin in a liquid or lozenge would be protective in the same way.

As we age, the production of saliva and the protective lactoferrin it contains decreases. This is one of the reasons that periodontal disease is so common. Lactoferrin in a liquid, lozenge or spray, or added to mouth rinse, tooth paste or other dental type product may be helpful to prevent problems associated with dry mouth.

Both human and bovine lactoferrin inhibited the adhesion of periodontitis-associated bacteria. The inhibitory effect was dose-dependent. (Alugupalli) Researchers at the University of Lund, Sweden, also demonstrated the binding effects of human lactoferrin on various bacterial strains associated with periodontal disease. (Kalfas)

Place a drop or two of colostrum-lactoferrin liquid directly on the affected area. The contents of colostrum-lactoferrin capsules can also be emptied, placing the powder directly on inflamed infected gum tissue.

Lactoferrin Inhibits Candida Albicans (Thrush)

A number of studies have demonstrated that bovine lactoferrin is able to inhibit the growth of Candida albicans. (Wakabayashi, Xu, Vorland) Japanese researchers showed that both human and bovine lactoferrin increased the action of neutrophils to inhibit Candida growth (Wakabayash) Chinese researchers demonstrated lactoferrin's inhibitory effect of Candida specifically in the oral ity. (Xu)

It is possible that topical applications could be cial as well for athletes foot, diaper rash, vagin other similar problems.

I am 75 years old and have been taking colostrum-lactoferrin lozenges for some time. It must be helping my immune system because I do not get the colds and flu viruses that everyone else around me seems to get. My whole family is taking the lozenges and none of them have been sick either.

But I think even more remarkable is the colostrum-lactoferrin spray. I had been experiencing inflammation and pain on the whole right side of my jaw for several months. It was very painful to chew. I was concerned that I was developing an abscess. I used one or two sprays a day for just two days and it was completely healed. It was unbelievable. I can't wait to tell my dentist as all he could recommend was to use salt water which did nothing. Everyone should know how wonderful colostrum-lactoferrin spray is!

Thank you, I.G.

I have been taking the colostrum lactoferrin lozenges for some time. Then I realized one d my gums were no longer bleeding when I w ing my teeth. This has been a problem I wa for quite a while, which is one of the early periodontal disease. I will keep taking the reason alone! Thank you, K.M

Diabetes

Insulin-like growth factor-I (IGF-I) can stimulate glucose utilization in nondiabetic subjects and that the action of the IGF-I receptor is normal in the skeletal muscle of patients with NIDDM, it seems possible that IGF-I might provide an e for the hyperglycemia of NIDDM. plasma levels of IGF-I in diabet those in either of the nondiabet

health problem as a dangerous, disease-causing bacteria. E. coli 0157:H7 causes bloody diarrhea (hemorrhagic colitis), hemolytic-uremic syndrome (a blood and kidney disease in children), and thrombotic thrombocytic purpura (a dire disease in the elderly). There is no specific treatment for E. coli infection.

In 1996, German researchers showed that components in colostrum from non-immunized cows effectively blocked the damaging effects of E. coli in humans. (Lissner)

In a placebo-controlled, double-blind study with individuals with E. coli-associated diarrhea, stool frequencies in the group treated with bovine colostrum were significantly reduced compared with those in the placebo group. No side effects were seen. (Huppertz)

Colostrum and lactoferrin are also effective against a number of other bacteria that are known to cause diarrhea.

Viruses: Colostrum has shown to be highly effective against many of the major diarrhea causing viruses including:rotavirus. In a double-blind, placebo-controlled trial, children with rotavirus diarrhea who orally received10 g. of bovine colostrum daily for 4 days experienced significant mprovement compared children who received a placebo. Clearance of rotavirus from the stool was also earlier in the colostrum group compared with the placebo group (average days, 1.5 vs. 2.9). No adverse reactions from the colostrum treatment were observed. (Sarker)

Parasites: Colostrum has shown to be highly effective against many of the major parasites including: C. parvum, Entamoeba histolytica (which causes ameobic dysentery), and Giardia lamblia (which causes malabsorption of fluids in the bowels and speeds contents through the intestines to produce diarrhea. By age 5, many children have acquired Giardia.)

Studies done on individuals with diarrhea who were otherwise healthy also show that supplemental bovine colostrum is very effective.

Fibromyalgia

A number of researchers have shown that fibromyalgia has clear signs of immune dysfunction. The results of a study conducted at the Department of Internal Medicine B, Carmel Medical Center, Haifa, Israel, suggest that there is a defect in the IL-2 pathway, which is related to protein kinase C activation in patients with fibromyalgia. (Hader)

Researchers in Spain at the Hospital University Virgen Del Rocio, showed that the number of T-cells expressing activation markers CD69 and CD25 is decreased in patients with fibromyalgia. The results suggest a defect in T cell activation. (Hernanz)

Studies on sleep disorders and the symptoms of fibromyalgia showed a link between IL-1, immune-neuroendocrine-thermal systems and the sleep-wake cycle which results in nonrestorative sleep, pain, fatigue, cognitive and mood symptoms in patients with fibromyalgia. (Moldofsky)

These studies all suggest fibromyalgia involves immune disregulation. Therefore, colostrum and it's regulatory factors such as lactoferrin could be of great benefits. Hopefully, there will be clinical trials conducted in the near future so this can be demonstrated.

Part of having fibromyalgia is that I seemed to get every cold and flu that came around. After I started taking the colostrum and lactoferrin lozenges I noticed that I didn't get sick as often and that I had more energy. When I did get sick, it didn't seem like I was sick as long as I normaly would be or as long as other people were. The lozenges also may be helping my irritable bowel problems that I have been struggling with for years. (T.M.)

Heart Disease

Plaque buildup involves free radical damage associated with oxidized LDL cholesterol caused by macrophage accumulation. Japanese researchers showed that supplemental bovine lactoferrin inhibits the accumulation of oxidized cholesterol in a dose-dependent manner and decreased oxidized cholesterol accumulation by more than 80% in humans.

Interestingly, the study showed that human lactoferrin was less potent than bovine lactoferrin. The results indicated that lactoferrin inhibits the binding of modified LDLs to macrophages, resulting in their loss of function. The results suggest that lactoferrin in the blood stream may act as an anti-atherogenic agent. (Kajikawa)

Lupus

Cytokine production of IL-6 and TNF-alpha is elevated in whole blood cell cultures of patients with SLE. (Swaak) Inflammatory cytokines are believed by the researchers to be in part responsible for problems associated with the condition. (Herrera-Esparza)

Because lactoferrin helps normalize production of both IL-6 and TNF-alpha, individuals with lupus may benefit greatly. Hopefully, clinical trials will soon demonstrate it's full potential. Colostrum and lactoferrin may also help support the immune system in general as individuals with lupus are at high risk for a variety of other health problems including periodontal disease, frequent colds and flu, etc.

Multiple Sclerosis (MS)

Research suggests that MS may be triggered by a viral infection. There is some preliminary research using orally administered hyper-immune colostrum on MS patients showing potential benefit as improvement was seen in some of the individuals. (Ebina)

Hyper-immune colostrum contains higher levels of antibodies than regular colostrum. I could not locate any studies using regular colostrum for MS so I can not compare the benefits. It is possible that regular colostrum may not be as effective as hyper-immune colostrum in this case; however, some studies have shown that regular colostrum is just as effective as hyper-immune for certain conditions. (Clark)

The risk of Diabetes (IDDM), H. pylori-related ulcers, Crohn's disease, and atopic disease is lower in individuals who were breast fed during infancy. These same protective factors apply to supplemental colostrum for adults and children.

Peptic Ulcer

Most ulcers are caused by the bacteria Helicobacter pylori (H. pylori). Many researchers have showed the benefits of bovine colostrum for ulcers caused by H. pylori. They show that bovine colostrum can block the binding of Helicobacter species to the lining of the stomach and intestinal tract therefore inhibit infection. (Bitzan, Falk, Hamosh, Wada)

Researchers at the University of Texas-Houston Medical School also found antibiotic properties of bovine lactoferrin against H. pylori and stated that lactoferrin should be further investigated for possible use in human H. pylori infections and peptic ulcers. (Dial)

Rheumatoid Arthritis

Elevated levels of IL-6 in synovial fluid appears to reflect the local proinflammatory, potentially erosive activity in rheumatoid arthritis. (Van Leeuwen. Brennan, Punzi)

Numerous studies, many conducted at the Institute of Immunology and Experimental Therapy, Polish Academy of Sciences, Weigla, Wroclaw, Poland, have been done to investigate the beneficial anti-inflammatory properties of orally ingested bovine lactoferrin.

Study results reveal an inhibition of the induced inflammation in the bovine lactoferrin-treated rats by 50%. The inhibition was also associated with a substantial decrease in IL-6 in the bovine lactoferrin-treated rats (94%). TNF-alpha production was also decreased, although to a lesser degree (48%). The researchers believed the decreased ability to produce inflammatory cytokines in bovine lactoferrin-treated rats may be the basis for the reduction in inflammation. (Zimecki)

Serum concentration of lactoferrin is also elevated in rheumatoid patients. Lactoferrin also diminishes the damaging effects of free radical release. Lactoferrin also controls the effector phase of cellular immune response and inhibits manifestations of autoimmune response in mice. (Adamik)

Weight Loss

Increasing levels of IGF-1 is also associated with weight loss as this and other growth factors found in colostrum help the body better utilize the food (especially glucose) you eat. Burning more glucose meaning less is stored and converted to fat.

IGF-1 levels decline as we grow older and also reduced by a lack of exercise, environmental toxins, stress and poor dietary habits. Supplemental colostrum can help restore IGF-1 levels and enhance metabolism, growth of lean muscle tissue and fat burning. Many people report that their appetite is better balanced when taking colostrum on a regular basis - that they experience less food cravings, and also experience loss of body fat.

BENEFITS FOR ATHLETES

For years athletes have been interested in colostrum because of the Insulin-like Growth Factor I and II (IGF-I and IGF-II) it contains. These are pro-insulin hormones that have anabolic (muscle promoting) effects. They are composed of an amino acid chain that resembles the hormone insulin.

Both bovine and human colostrum growth factors have demonstrated the ability to stimulate protein synthesis and inhibit protein degradation. (Francis, Rinderkneckt, Humbel) IGF-1 in bovine colostrum contains the identical amino acid sequence except for a 26 amino acid segment on the front of the bovine molecule which, when split by digestive acids in our stomach, releases a highest concentrations of IGF-I available in nature.

The primary function of IGF-1 and II in colostrum is to promote rapid tissue growth through protein synthesis of the newborn. In adults, IGF-1 and IGF-II are important factors involved in cell proliferation and metabolism, regulation of tissue repair, growth and differentiation. Remember that our tissues are in a constant state of repair.

IGF-1 assists cells toward cell division and the ability to complete DNA synthesis. IGF-1 not only helps cell growth by division, but also by enhancing cell specialization. IGF-1 communicates an anabolic signal to cells, regulating cell division and differentiation as the muscle acquires an increased need for strength or as injury to the muscle is incurred. IGF-1 promotes the growth of muscle and bone.

IGF-1 is believed to bring aging, resting cells back into a balanced state optimizing cell activity and tissue performance.

The following are associated with IGF-1:

- Increased physical performance
- Increased mental performance
- Increased physical endurance
- Increase in lean muscle tissue growth
- Wound healing and repair

Many colostrum users report decreased recovery time and decreased soreness after acute exercise when using a colostrum supplement. This is, of course subjective, but there is some scientific evidence that support these claims.

Anabolic and tissue repair functions of insulin-like growth factors have been studied extensively, and it seems that healing of injuries and post-workout recovery are improved as well with IGF-1 supplementation.

Obviously the anti-inflammatory benefits of colostrum/lactoferrin are of great interest to the athlete, but increased nutrient absorption is also of significance. IGF-1 is also important for its affect on development, diabetes and other chronic diseases.

Finnish Olympic Ski Team members supplementing colostrum confirm its athletic benefits. Blood creatine-kinase levels were measured over a seven-day period of heavy training. Creatine-kinase is a critically important muscle cell enzyme that acts as a marker for muscle-cell damage. When creatine-kinase levels rise in the blood, there probably has been muscle-cell damage. Compared to ski team members who drank placebos, the athletes who drank a colostrum beverage showed one-half the blood creatine-kinase levels after four days. The individuals in the colostrum supplementation group also reported that they felt better and felt that their performance was improving. The researchers theorize that IGF-I in colostrum could encourage muscle cells to repair themselves more quickly after stress from intense exercise. (Anderson)

THERAPEUTIC RECOMMENDATIONS

Excellent quality colostrum liquid can be effectively used for severely immuno-compromised individuals. Therapeutic doses of an excellent quality colostrum liquid are as follows:

First 10 days: *1 Tablespoon 3 times per day*

Next 10 days: *1 Tablespoon 2 times per day*

Next 30 days: *1 Tablespoon 1 time per day/reevaluate*

The above regime is for excellent quality colostrum liquid only. Moderate or poor quality colostrum may require more and will have unpredictable results.

The fat and casein are removed in liquid colostrum. As a result, the levels of some of the components, such as PRP, are of a higher concentration. This important, powerful regulatory Proline-Rich-Polypeptide is very important for individuals with debilitating conditions.

While the many important effects of PRP are beyond the scope of this book, I do however, want to point out one very interesting Polish study I came across on Alzheimer's Disease.

In a 12-month, double-blind trial with a PRP complex isolated from colostrum (orally delivered), 8 of 15 Alzheimer's patients improved. In the 7 others the disease stabilized. In contrast, none of the 31 patients receiving selenium or a placebo with similar mild or moderate Alzheimer's improved. The results obtained showed that PRP improves the outcome of Alzheimer's patients with mild to moderate dementia. (Leszek)

TOPICAL USE FOR COLOSTRUM-LACTOFERRIN

It is not surprising that colostrum and lactoferrin are also available in topical application products such as creams. There is not yet much published research on this mode of application, but the potential for benefits definitely exists.

There are many reports that colostrum taken internally is beneficial for skin conditions such as hives and eczema. This, of course, makes perfect sense as these conditions are often allergy related. Anti-inflammatory properties and regulatory factors in colostrum and lactoferrin could be very beneficial.

Tryptase is found in high levels in mast cells in individuals with psoriasis (Harvima), eczema and dermatitis. (Welle, Jarvikallio) Because lactoferrin is known to have an inhibitory effect against tryptase, it is possible that either oral or topical applications would be very beneficial.

Antibiotic and antiviral properties make colostrum and lactoferrin an excellent treatment for various wounds, infections (possibly acne), etc. Epithelial growth factors can help speed healing while anti-inflammatory factors help reduce swelling.

We know that topical applications from colostrum liquid, lozenges or making a paste out of powder and a small amount of water are highly beneficial for periodontal problems.

CHOOSING A COLOSTRUM-LACTOFERRIN DIETARY SUPPLEMENT

It is easy to get confused when examining the marketing literature produced by so many companies selling colostrum. Colostrum marketing has been covered in numerous trade and consumer journals and television programs. The following information will be useful to separate fact from fiction and to obtain the best quality product that ultimately lead to the best results for you and your family.

Quality, purity, efficacy, delivery system and price are all important factors in choosing any dietary supplement. The following are the major points you want to consider when selecting a colostrum/lactoferrin supplement:

1. Quality and potency of colostrum and lactoferrin

2. Delivery system

3. Reputation of manufacture

Quality and Potency

Because colostrum and lactoferrin are bioactive, the quality can vary widely from providers. This causes the selection process to be more difficult. To manufacture colostrum, tremendous care must be used in the collection, purification, processing and storage. Colostrum's efficacy is contingent upon the following:

Collection

As a liquid, cow's milk contains approximately 4% protein (80% casein and only 10% immunoglobulins). At birth, colostrum contains almost 20% protein, yet quickly degrades to just 4% in 24 hours. Approximately 55% of this is immunoglobulins.

When colostrum is properly harvested and dried, it should contain at least 50% protein. Immunoglobulins will then be at least 40% of the protein content.

Typically this will require milking within the first 6 hours after birth. Subsequent milkings contain transitional milk which if blended with the first milking, compromise the delicate balance of immunofactors in the colostrum. Refer to the chart on page 18 to see how quickly the composition changes after the birth of the calf.

In 1913 the USDH defined colostrum as the milk collected in the first six milkings after partration. This definition was created to prevent colostrum and transitional milk from being sold as milk for human consumption - not to define true colostrum to be used for human immune enhancement–which was unheard of almost 90 years ago.

What this means is that some "so-called colostrum" on the market is not colostrum at all, but actually a whey protein concentrate (WPC). Whey protein concentrate has a very different composition than true colostrum. Only a small amount of true excellent quality colostrum is required to activate an immune system response in the body. Much larger quantities are required from WPC, 3 grams or more daily. At this level, quantities of IGF-1 should be high enough to have a beneficial effect.

After the colostrum is collected it should be frozen and transferred to a processing facility where the fluid is dried under conditions that do not alter or destroy any of its many special components.

- Source of the dairy herd
- Practices of the dairy farmer
- Collection time (optimal: 3-6 hours after delivery)
- Storage and handling of the raw colostrum

Purification

All colostrum raw materials must be tested to be certified free of pathogenic microorganisms. Products should be coded with a lot number that corresponds to laboratory test results.

- Pasteurization techniques
- Whether or not the pasteurized colostrum is modified by removing any: lactose, fat. casein or other component.

Processing

Temperatures used to process colostrum should not be above 105 degrees F. in order to preserve its special immune components. At 106 degrees F., enzymes breakdown.

- Spray drying or freeze-drying
- Storage of the dried colostrum
- Processing into liquid, lozenges, capsules or left
  in powder form

Storage

Some colostrum products may require refrigeration to maintain freshness and optimal shelf life.

- Care in handling and storage by the manufacturer and retailer

Source of the Dairy Herd

Seek a source of colostrum that is in the same geographic location that you currently live in. In other words, if you live in Europe obtain European colostrum. In Asia obtain Asian colostrum. If you live in the United States, obtain U.S. colostrum. The reason is that "local" colostrum is more likely to offer protection against "local" strains of infectious microorganisms.

Healthy Cattle

Colostrum should come from disease-free herds, in other words - healthy cattle. In the US, they should be Grade A dairy cattle. Dairy cattle, as a general rule, are typically healthier in smaller, closely supervised herds. An average herd size of fifty or so cattle in a family farm are more closely watched, cared for and supervised than a herd of thousands or more. Why? Simple logic. When a farm family makes their living from fifty mature dairy cattle, each cow has a name, a history, and is personally cared for twice a day by the family.

In large herds, employees are hired to care for the animals and the employee's paycheck comes whether or not the herd is carefully watched over or not. It becomes big business and the personal touch...and care are no longer important.

Drug-Free Cattle

Colostrum from cattle raised without exposure to antibiotics, pesticides, and hormones is preferred. These drugs stress and disrupt the normal homeostatic balance in the body.

Antibiotics: The United States produces over 50 million tons of antibiotics annually. Half of these are used for export and the other 25 million tons are given to animals. Most veterinarians use standard antibiotics. U.S. dairy farmers are much more conscious of the fact that whatever they put into their herd will in turn come out in the milk they drink.

Pesticides: Pesticides are widely used in numerous countries in the world. Regardless of the geographic location of the dairy herds, independent assays should be performed on each lot of colostrum to prove safety. If levels are below the standards set for safety, daily use of colostrum will not pose a health threat. Of course, the smallest amount of quality colostrum will yield the least amount of toxins.

It is very difficult to find anything that is 100% pesticide free as residues can be detected in the soil from pesticide use from many decades ago. Feed grown in these soils may contain minute traces of residue even through the farming practice today may be truly "100% organic." Be wary of those who claim "100% pesticide free" - it is not likely unless they brought it in from the moon!

Hormones: Hormones are of two major types: growth and milk production hormones.

Growth hormones are given to young animals in the beef, pork and poultry industries to increase the amount of meat per animal. These hormones are rarely, if ever, given to the animals in a dairy herd.

Milk production hormones cannot be given to a pregnant dairy cow. If the pregnant cow is given milk hormones, she will abort the calf and therefore not produce colostrum. True colostrum is produced by the mother cow prior to giving birth and by definition cannot contain milk production hormones.

Delivery System

Colostrum and lactoferrin products are available as powders in capsules, tablets, chewables, lozenges, as a food additive and in various formulas. Colostrum is also available as a pure liquid, without spray-   drying. Creams for topical use containing colostrum and lactoferrin are also available.

Scientific studies with the greatest benefit to the test groups are achieved with the oral delivery of high quality colostrum. Oral delivery means absorption in the mouth, such as sublingually (under the tongue) or slowly dissolving a lozenge. Swallowing hard pressed caplets or capsules is not a true mucosal delivery.

Your delivery decision should also be based upon its

intended end use. If you only want to treat the mouth and gums such as in the case of an abcess or periodontal disease, a liquid or powder applied directly to the affect area is likely to be your best choice, although lozenges would work as well. If you are looking to supplement your infants' bottle, then you need a liquid. If you want to treat systemic conditions such as lupus, diabetes, arthritis, asthma, etc., then you need a good mucosal delivery system such as a lozenge.

Reputation of Manufacture

Beware of manufacturers who cut colostrum with whey protein, which has lower levels of immunoglobulins and other important factors. The manufacturer's independent certifications should show the following:

	Colostrum	**Whey**
Lactose concentration	Very low	Yes
Lactalbumin (a potentially allergenic protein)	None	Yes
IGF-1 content	High	Low
Lactoferrin	High	Low
Immunoglobulins	High	Low
Glycoproteins	High	Low

Be Wary Of False Advertising

Marketing colostrum has become a big business. If you try a certain brand of colostrum and it does not work, don't give up on colostrum. Instead try a different brand, a different form of delivery or both. Remember that many colostrum studies are performed by delivering the colostrum directly into the oral cavity. Capsule delivery of colostrum is likely to not have the same result.

Some of the false advertising surrounding colostrum include the following:

1. *Colostrum is the milk-like fluid produced by all female mammals in the first 24 to 36 hours directly after giving birth. It lasts until the onset of lactation, which occurs within 36 to 72 hours post-partum.* **False.** True colostrum is only attained in the first milking after giving birth. After 24 hours, the colostrum is less than one-forth the quality it should be. This would then require a suggested use of more than four times the amount. The sooner it is collected after birth (preferably 3 to 6 hours), the more efficacious it is.

2. *You can obtain raw colostrum from a dairy farmer.* **False.** The USDA prohibits the sale of raw, unpasteurized colostrum for human use.

3. *If colostrum is frozen, it becomes insoluble in water.* **False**. If colostrum is soluble in water as a liquid, it cannot be rendered insoluble merely by freezing and then thawing. In fact, when colostrum is frozen after harvesting, it will retain its bioactivity longer and will resist the chemical changes that eventually will occur.

4. *Lozenges and tablets are processed using high heat and therefore are ineffective.* **False**. Experienced manufacturers know that cold-pressed lozenges and tablets are not made with high heat. Lozenges and tablets are the preferred method of taking colostrum, so encapsulators generate unfavorable press to make their product more attractive.

5. *Liquid colostrum is not as good as capsules.* **False.** For the same reasons above.

6. *Colostrum should be de-fatted.* **False.** Many of the immuno-factors found in colostrum are contained in the fat. Also, the de-fatting process degrades the colostrum even further.

7. *Colostrum should be de-lactosed.* **False.** Every time colostrum is further processed or an element removed, the colostrum is compromised.

8. *Colostrum is safe for lactose-intolerant individuals.* **Generally false.** The greater the amount of time between birth and collection the greater the lactose content so it depends on the quality of the colostrum. Over 77 mg. lactose will invoke a response in lactose intolerant individuals.

9. *You must take 2 to 4 grams of colostrum daily to receive benefits.* **False.** Just 125 mg. of high quality colostrum taken orally will produce an immune system response.

10. *There is not a good source of colostrum in the United States.* **False.** The United States has several good or excellent providers of colostrum. Also keep in mind that "local" colostrum is preferable.

These are just a few of the false advertising techniques used by unscrupulous manufacturers to promote their product. Read, analyze, ask and try the product. If it doesn't work, try another manufacturer and another form of delivery.

BIBLIOGRAPHY

Aabakken. Lam.; short term effect of bovine colostrum in patients with throat angina. A placebo controlled study. Statistical Report No. 309, Vuramed, Norway. Norges Apatekares tidsskritt, 98 nr 22. April 1990.

Acosta-Altaxuirano. c. et al. 1987. Antiamoebic properties of human colostrum. Adv. Exp. Med. Biol. 216B:1347-52.

Adamik B; Wlaszczyk A d.actoferiin--ita role in defense against infection and Immunotropic properties, Katedra I Elinika Añesteziologli I Inlensywnej Terapli Akademli Medyeniej we Wroclawiu. Postepy Hig Med Dosw 1996;50(1):33-41:

Adamik B; Zimecki M; Wlaszczyk A;et al; Lactoferrin effects on the in vitro immune response in critically ill patients. Dept. of Anesthesiology and Intensive Therapy, U. Medical School, Wroclaw, Poland. Arch Immunol Ther Exp (Warsz) 1998; 46(3): 169-76.

Adamik B; Wlaszczyk A; Lactoferrin--its role in defense against infection and Immunotropic properties, Katedra i Klinika Añesteziologii i Intensywnej Terapii Akademii Medycznej we Wroclawiu. Postepy Hig Med Dosw 1996;50(1):33-41.

Adeyemi EO; Campos LB; Lolzou S; et al; Plasma dactoferrin and neutrophil elastase in rheumatoid arthritis and systemic lupus erythematosus Dept of Medicine. Royal Postgraduate Medical School, Hammeramith Hospital, London. Br J Rheumatol 1990 Feb:29(1):15-20.

Alugupalli KR; Kalfas S; Inhibitory effects of lactoferrin on the adhesion of Actinobacillus actinomycetemcomitans and Prevotella intermedia to fibroblasts and epithelial cells. Dept of Oral Microbiology, Malmo General Hospital, Lund University, Sweden. APMIS 1995 Feb; 103(2): 154-60.

Amini HR; Ascencio F; Ruiz-Bustos E; Romero MJ; Wadstrom T; Cryptic domains of a 60 kDa heat shock protein of Helicobacter pylori bound to bovine lactoferrin. Department of Medical Microbiology, U of Lund, Sweden. FEMS Immuniol Med Microbiol 1996 Dec 31;16(3-4):247-55.

Anderson, 0:; Running Research News. pp 11. January-February, 1994.

Arao S; Matsuura S; Nonomura M; Miki K; Kabasawa K Nakanishi H: Measurement of urinary lactoferrin as a marker of urinary tract infection. Planning and Development Division, Iatron Laboratories, Inc., 1-11-4, Higashikanda, Chiyoda-ku, Tokyo, Japan. J Clin Microbiol 1999 Mar; 37(3):553-7.

Atlinson JC; Yeh C; Oppenhelm FG: et al; Elevation of sallvaiy antimicrobial proteins following HIV- I infection. Clinical Investigations and Patient Care Branch, National Institute of Dental Research, Bethesda, Maiyland. J Acquir Immune Defic Syndr 1990:3(l):4d-8.

Baldwin, Tom. et alp: Elevation of intracedullar free calcium levels In HEp-2 cells infected with enteropathogenic Eseherichia coll. Infection and immunity. (May 1991) p. 1599-1604.

Ballard, J.F.. Cl ad.; The Relationship Between the Insulin Content and Inhibitory Effects of Bovine Codostrum on Protein Breakdown in Cultored Cells. Journal of Cellular Physiology (1982) Vol.110,249-254.

Ballard FJ; Nield MK Frands GL Knowles sE; Regulation of Intracellular protein degradation by insulin and growth factors. Acta Blod Med Ger 1981:40(10-11):1293-300.

Bauxurucker CR Blum JW; Effects of dietary reeomkinant human Insulin-like growth factor-I on concentrations of honnones and growth factees in the blood of newborn calves. J Exxloalfhod 1994 Jan. 140(l):15-21.

Bayard BL James MA; Hyperimmune bovine colostmin inefficacious as multiple sclerosis therapy in double-blind study. Department of Food and Nutiltion, University of Wiseonslnstout. Menomonie. J Am Diet Assoc 1987 Oct87(d0): 1388-90.

Baynes RD; Bezwoda WR; Mansoor N; Neutrophil lactoferrin content in viral infections. Am J Clin Pathol 1988 Feb;89(2):225-8.

Ben-Aryeh H, et al, Oral health and salivary composition in diabetic patients. J Diabetes Complications. 1993 Jan-Mar;7(1):57-62.

Bereket A; Lang CH; Wilson TA; Alterations in the growth hormone-insulin-like growth factor axis in insulin dependent diabetes mellitus. Horm Metab Res 1999 Feb-Mar;31(2-3):172-81.

Bertotto A Castellucci G; RadlclOrbi M; Bartolucci M: Vaccaro R, CD4O ligand expression on the surface of colostral T cells. Department of Paediatrics. Perugia Universlty Medical School. Italy. Arch Dis Child Fetal Neonatal Ed 1996 Mar. 74(21:F135-6.

Bessler H: Straussberg R Hart J: NoW I: Sirota L; Human codostnrm stimulates cytodine production. Hematology and Immunology Research Laboratory, Golda Medical Center, Hashan,n Hospital. Petah-Tiqva. Israel. Biod Neonate 1996:69(6):376-82.

Bezault J; Ilhimani R, Wiprovnick J; Furmanaki P: Human lactoferrin Inhibits growth of solid tumors and development of experimental metastases in mice. New York University, Department of Biology. New York 10003. Cancer Res 1994 May 1,54(91:2310-2.

Bitman J: Hamosh M; Hamosh P: Lutes V; Neville MC; Seacat J; Wood DL; Milk composition and volume during the Onset of lactation in a diabetic mother. Am J Chin Nutr 1989 Dec;50(6): 1364-9.

Bitzan MM; Gold BD; Philpott DJ; et al; Inhibition of Helicobacter pylori and Helicobacter mustelae binding to lipid receptors by bovine colostrum. J Infect Dis 1998 Apr;177(4):955-61.

Bouda, J.. et ad.; Vitamins A and Carotene Metabolism in Cows and their Calves Fed From Buckets. ACTA Vet. Brno. (1980) Vol.49(1-21.45-52.

Bouda. J., et ad.; Vitamins E and C in the Blood Plasma of Cows and their Calves Fed lmm Buckets. ACTA Vet. Bnio. (1980) Vol.49(1-2). 53-58.

Brsmdtzaeq, Per-, The Secretory Immune System of Lactating Human Mammary Gland Compared with other Exoezine Organs. Annals of N.Y. Academy of Science (1983) Vol 409, 353-378.

Bramdtaaeg. P. Annals of the N.Y. Academy of sclerceoo (1983) Vol.409353-378.

Brennan FM, et al. Detection of interleukin 8 biological activity in synovial fluids from patients with rheumatoid arthritis and production of interleukin 8 mRNA by isolated synovial cells. Eur J Immunol. 1990 Sep;20(9):2141-4.

Brock JH; Ismail M: Sanchez L; Interaction of lactoferrin with mononuclear and colon carcinoma cells. University Department of Immunology, Western Infirmary. Glasgow, Scotland. United Kingdom. Mv Exp Med Biol 1994; 357:157-69.

Brock, J. (1995). Lactoferrin: a multifunctional immunoregulatory protein? Immunology Today. 16,9: 417-419.

Brown DL; Kane CD; Chernausek SD; Greenhaigh DG; Differential expression and localization of insulin-like growth factors I and II in cutaneous wounds of diabetic and nondiabetic mice. Am J Pathol 1997 Sep;151(3):715-24.

Buescher ES: The effects of colostrum or neutrophil function: decreased deformability with increased cytoskeletom-associated actir. Adv Exp Med Biol 1991:310:131-6.

Bucacher ES; Medlheran SM: Antioxidant properties of human colostrum. Department of Pedlatiles, University of Texas Medical School, Houston 77030. Pedlair Res 1988 Jul:24(1l:14-9.

Buescher ES: The effects of colostrum on neutrophil function: decreased deformability with increased cytoskeletor-associated actir. Mv Exp Med Biod 1991:310:131-6.

Buescher ES: Meldheran SM: Frenck RW: Further characterization of human codostrad antioxidants: identification of an ascorbate-like element as an antioxidant component and demonstmtior of antioxidant heterogeneity. Pedlair Res 1989 Mar,25(3):266-70.

Bueseher. ES. and Meliheran, S.M. 1988. Antioxidant properties of human colostrum. Pedlat. Res. 24:14-19.

Buhler C; Hammon H; et al; Small intestinal morphology in eight-day-old calves fed colostrum for different durations or only milk replacer and treated with long-R3- insulin-like growth factor I and growth hormone. J Anim Sci 1998 Mar;76(3):758-65.

Burke, Edmund. Colostrum as an athletic enhancer and help for AIDS, Nutrition Science News, May 1996. 30-32.

Butte NF; Wong WW; Fiorotto M; Smith EO; Garza C Influence of early feeding mode on body composition of infants. USDA/ARS Children' Nutrition Research Center. Baylor College of Medicine. Houston. Tex.' USA. Biol Neonate 1995:67(61:414-24.

Cameron CM; Kostyo JL, Adamaflo NA; et al; The acute effects of growlln hormone or amino acid transport and protein synthesis are due to its Insulir-like action. Ann Arbor 48109-0622. Endocrinology 1988 Feb; 122(21:471-4.

Carlson SE. Arachidonic acid status of human infants: influence of gestational age at birth and diets with very long chain n-3 and n-6 fatty acids. J Nutr 1996 Apr;126(4 Suppl):f092S-8S.

Chase, CCL.. et al. 1995. mt effects of oralantibiotic therapies on immune function and productivity. Proc. Am. Assoc. Swine Pract. 26:111-14.

Christensen, Knud. et ad.;: Colostrum treatment of HIV infected patients with oral pseudomembranous candida infection. European Conference on Clinical Aspects of HIV Infection. Brussels, December 1987.

Close, M. J., Howlett, A. R. Roskelley, C. D. Desprez, P. Y., et al; Division of Life Sciences, Berkeley National Laboratory. University of California, Berkeley, CA' October 30, 1997.

Cockburn, F;, Neonatal brain and dietary lipids, Archieves of Disease in Childhood, 1994, 70 F1-F2.

Cortizo AM; Lee PD; Cedola NV; Jasper H; Gagliardino JJ; Relationship between non-enzymatic glycosylation and changes in serum insulin-like growth factor-1 (IGF-1) and IGF-binding protein-3 levels in patients with type 2 diabetes mellitus. Acta Diabetol 1998 Jul;35(2):85-90.

Cregar L; Elrod KC; Putnam D; Moore WR; Neutrophil myeloperoxidase is a potent and selective inhibitor of mast cell tryptase. Departments of Biochemistry and Enzymology, Axys Pharmaceuticals, Inc., South San Francisco, California, Arch Biochem Biophys 1999 Jun 1;366(1):125-30.

Crime Thnes, Vol 2, No. 1, 1986. Mother's Milk increases IQ, reduces neurological problems" The Wacker Foundation, Dept. 132. 1106 North Gflbert Road, Suite 2, Mesa, AZ 85203.

Da Dalt S: Moncada A Priori N, Valesini G; Pivetti-Pemi P: The lactoferrin tear test in the diagnosis of S.Jogren's syndrome. Institute of Ophthalmology, University of Roma La Sapienza, Italy. Eur J Ophthalmol 1996 Jul-Sep:6(3):284-6.

Damiens E; El Yazidi I; et al; Role of heparan sulphate proteoglycans in the regulation of humanlactoferrin binding and activity in the MDA-MB-231 breast cancer cell line. Eur J Cell Biol 1998 Dec;77(4):344-51.

Damiens E; Mazurier J; el Yazidi I; Masson M Duthille I; Spik G; Boilly-Marer Y; Effects of human lactoferrin on NK cell cytotoxicity against haematopoietic and epithelial tumour cells. Biochim Biophys Acta 1998 Apr 24;1402(3):277-87.

Dax-wish: Compaxitive Study of Breat Milk of Mothers Deliverylng Preterm and Term Infants- Protein, Fat. and Lactose. Nabnmg. Vol. 33, No. 3 (1989): p. 249.

Defer MC: Dugas B: Picard 0: Damais C: Impairment of circulating lactoferrin in HIV- 1 infection. U313 INSERM, Centre de Recherche des Cordeliers, Paris, France. Cell Mol Biol (Nolsy-le-grand) 1995 May;41(3):417-2159.

Dhaenens L; Szczebara F; Van Nieuwenhuyse S; Husson MO; Comparison of iron uptake in different Helicobacter species. Laboratoire de bacteriologie-hygiene, faculte de medecine Henri- Warembourg, Lille, France. Res Microbiol 1999 Sep;150(7):475-81.

Dohm GL; Elton CW; Raju MS; Mooney ND; et al; IGF-I--stimulated glucose transport in human skeletal muscle and IGF-I resistance in obesity and NIDDM. Diabetes 1990 Aug;39(9):1028-32.

Dial EJ; Hall LR; Serna H; Romero JJ; Fox JG; Lichtenberger LM; Antibiotic properties of bovine lactoferrin on Helicobacter pylori. Department of Integrative Biology, The University of Texas-Houston Medical School. Dig Dis Sci 1998 Dec;43(12):2750-6.

Di Biase N; Napoli A; Caiola S; Buongiorno AM; et al; IGF-1 levels in diabetic pregnant women and their infants. Ann Ist Super Sanita 1997;33(3):379-82.

Dunger DB; Acerini CL; IGF-I and diabetes in adolescence. Diabetes Metab 1998 Apr;24(2):101-7.

Di Poi E, et alIL-6 and some natural inhibitors of chronic human inflammation in RA and SLE. Clin Exp Rheumatol. 1999 Jul-Aug;17(4):513.

Ebina T: Sate A Umezu K, Am H: Ishida N: Seki H: Tsukamoto T: 'dYeatment of multiple sclerosis with anti-measles cow codostrum. Med Microbiol Immunol (Berl) 1984:173(2):87-93.

Ebina, T., et al.; Prevention of rotavlrus infection with cow colostrum containing antibody against human rotavirus. The Lancet. 1983; 29:1029-30.

Ebina T: Ohta M: Kanamaru Y: Yamamoto-Osumi Y: Baba K: Passive immunizations of suckling mice and infants with bovine colostrum containing antibodies to human rotavirus. J Med Virol 1992 Oct;38(2):117-23.

Ebina T: Sato A Umezu K Ishida N: Ohyama 5: Olzumi A Aikawa K Katagiri 5: Katsushima N: Imal A et ad: Prevention of rotavirus infection by oral administration of cow codostrum containing antihumanrotavirus antibody. Med Microbiol Immunod (Berl) 1985:174(4): 177-85.

Elrod KC; Moore WR; Abraham WM; Tanaka RD; Lactoferrin, a potent tryptase inhibitor, abolishes late-phase airway responses in allergic sheep. Arris Pharmaceutical Corporation, South San Francisco, California. Am J Respir Crit Care Med 1997 Aug;156(2 Pt 1):375-81.

Enestrom S; Bengtsson A; Frodin TDermal IgG deposits and increase of mast cells in patients with fibromyalgia—relevant findings or epiphenomena? Scand J Rheumatol 1997;26(4):308-13.

Falk P; Roth KA; Boren T; Westblom TU; et al: An in vitro adherence assay reveals that Helicobacter pylori exhibits cell lineage-specific tropism in the human gastric epithelium. Proc Natl Acad Sci U SA; 1993 Mar 1;90(5):2035-9.

Fergusson, DM, Beautrais, AL, Silva, PA, Breast-feeding and cognitive development in the first seven years of life. Soc Sci Med 1982, Vol 16, pp 1705-1708.

Fleener, Scott, Journal of Dairy Science, Vol. 63, Nov. 1980.

Francis, Geofty, Upton, Faye, et al.: Insulin-like growth factors 1 and 2 in bovine colostrum. Biochem J. 1988. 251: 95-103.

Goke B; Fehmann HC; Insulin and insulin-like growth factor-I: their role as risk factors in the development of diabetic cardiovascular disease. Diabetes Res Clin Pract 1996 Feb;30 Suppl:93-106.

Goldman, A and R. Goldhlum: "Human Milk: Imunologic-Nutiritonal Relationship" Micronutrients and Immune Functions, Annals of the New York Academy of Science, Vol. 587(1990] pg 238-243.

Grazioso CF; Buescher ES: Inhibition of neutrophil function by human milk. Cell Immunol 1996 Mar 15:168(21:125-32.

Greenberg PD; Cello JP: Treatment of severe dian'hea caused by Cxypto-sporidium parvum with oral bovine immunoglobulin concentrate in patients with AIDS. J Acquir Immune Defic Syndr Hum Retrovirol 1996 Dec 1:13(41:348-54.

Groenink J; Walgreen-Weterings E; et al; Cationic amphipathic peptides, derived from bovine and human lactoferrin, with antimicrobial activity against oral pathogens. FEMS Microbiol Lett 1999 Oct 15;179(2):217-22.

Grosvenor CE: Picciano MF; Baumrucker CR Hormones and growth factors In milk Pennsylvania State University, University Park 16802. Endocr Rev 1993 Dec: 14(61:710-28.

Gulve EA, Dice JF: Regulation of protein synthesis and degradation in L8 myotubes. Effects of serum, insulin and insulin-like growth factors. Harvard Medical School, Boston, Blochem J 1989 Jun 1:260(21:377-87.

Hader N; Rimon D; ey al; Altered interleukin-2 secretion in patients with primary fibromyalgia syndrome. Department of Internal Medicine B, Carmel Medical Center, Halfa, Israel. Arthritis Rheum 1991 Jul;34(7):866-72.

Hadorn U, et al. Delaying colostrum intake by one day has important effects on metabolic traits and on gastrointestinal and metabolic hormones in neonatal calves. J Nutr. 1997 Oct;127(10):2011-23.

69

Hadsell DL: Baumrucker CR Kenslnger RS Effecis of elevated blood Insulin-like growth factor-I (IGF-1) concenlmtion upon IGF-1 in bovine marnmary secretions during the rolostrum phase. J Endocrinol 1993 May; 137(21:223-30.

Hanson LA; Mattsby-Baltzer I; Engberg I; Roseanu A; et al: Anti-inflammatory capacities of human milk: lactoferrin and secretory IgA inhibit endotoxin-induced cytokine release. Dept. of Clinical Immunology, U of Goteborg, Sweden. Adv Exp Med Biol 1995;371A:669-72.

Hanson, et al: "Mucosal Immunity" Annals of N.Y. Academy of Science, (1983) Vol 409. 15.

Harmsen MC: Swart PJ: de Bethune MP: et al.: Antiviral effects of plasma and milk proteins: lactoferrin showspotert activity against both human immunodeficiency virus and human cytomegalovirus replication in vim. J Infect Dia 1995 Aug: 172(21:380-8.

Harper, J.M.M., Soar, J.B., and Buttery. J.P.: "Changes in protein metabolism of ovine primary muscle cultores on treatment of growth hornone. insulln. insulln-like growth facto: I or epidermad growth factor.: J Endocrinology 1987, 112: 87-96.

Harvima IT; Haapanen L; Ackermann L; Naukkarinen A; Harvima RJ; Horsmanheimo MDecreased chymase activity is associated with increased levels of protease inhibitors in mast cells of psoriatic lesions. Department of Dermatology. Kuopio University Hospital, Finland. Acta Derm Venereol 1999 Mar;79(2):98-104.

Hasegawa K; Motsuchi W; Tanaka S; Inhibition with lactoferrin of in vitro infection with human herpes virus. Jpn J Med Sci Biol 1994 Apr;47(2):73-85.

Heinz-Erian P; Achmuller M; et al: Vitamin C concentrations in maternal plasma, amniotic fluid, umbilical cord blood, the plasma of newborn infants, colostrum and transitory and mature breast milk. Padiatr Padol 1987;22(2):163-78.

Hennlngs, J., et al. 1993. Inimunocoropromlse In gnotobiotic pigs induced h verotoxin-producing Escherichla colt (0111 NM). Infect. Immun. 61:23048.

Hernanz W; Valenzuela A; Quijada J; et al: ;Lymphocyte subpopulations in patients with primary fibromyalgia. J Rheumatol 1994 Nov;21(11):2122-4.

Herrera-Esparza R; Barbosa-Cisneros O; Villalobos- Hurtado R; Avalos-Diaz E; Renal expression of IL-6 and TNF-alpha genes in lupus nephritis. Lupus 1998;7(3):154-8.

Ho. P.C.. Lawton. John. W.M: "Human Codostral Cells: Phagocytosis and Killing of E. Coli and C. Albicans" Infection and immunity (1978) Vol 13, 1433.

Hooton JW; Pabst HF: Spady DW: Paetkau V: Human codosinim contains an activity that inhibits the production of IL-2. Department of Biochemistry, Walter MacKenzie Center, University of Alberta, Edmonton, Canada. Clin Exp Immunol 1991 Oct:86(3):520-4.

Huppertz HI; Rutkowski S; Busch DH; Lissner R; et al: Bovine colostrum ameliorates diarrhea in infection with diarrheagenic Escherichia coli, shiga toxin-producing E. Coli, and E. coli expressing intiminand hemolysin. J Pediatr Gastroenterol Nutr 1999 Oct;29(4):452-6.'

Hurdey WL; Hegarty HM: Melzder JT In vim inhibition of mammaly cell growth by lactoferrin: a comparative study. Life Sci 1994:55(241:1955-63.

Huxley, Dj.. et al. 1995. Evidence supporting the mechanism of enteric protection provided the colostrad wheyed supplements. Proc. Am. Assoc. Bovine Pract. 27:1938.

Ishiguro Y; Mucosal proinflammatory cytokine production correlates with endoscopic activity of ulcerative colitis." J Gastroenterol 1999 Feb;34(1):66-74.

Itoh Y; Igarashi T; Tatsuma N; et al; Autoimmune fatigue syndrome and fibromyalgia syndrome. Nippon Ika Daigaku Zasshi 1999 Aug;66(4):239-44.

Jara LJ; Lavalle C; Fraga A; et al; Prolactin, immunoregulation, and autoimmune diseases. Semin Arthritis Rheum 1991 Apr;20(5):273-84.

Jarvikallio A; Naukkarinen A; Harvima IT; et al:Quantitative analysis of tryptase- and chymase-containing mast cells in atopic dermatitis and nummular eczema. Br J Dermatol 1997 Jun;136(6):871-7.

Jones BM; Kwok CC; Kung AW; Effect of radioactive iodine therapy on cytokine production in Graves' disease: transient increases in interleukin-4 (IL-4), IL-6, IL-10, and tumor necrosis factor-alpha, with longer term increases in interferon- gamma production. J Clin Endocrinol Metab 1999 Nov;84(11):4106-10.

Juto, P.: Human Milk Stimulates B-Cell Function. Archives of Diseases in Childhood. Vol 60, no 7(1985) pg 610-613.

Kajikawa M; Ohta T; Takase M; et al; Lactoferrin inhibits cholesterol accumulation in macrophages mediated by acetylated or oxidized low-density lipoproteins. Biochim Biophys Acta 1994 Jun 23;1213(1):82-90.

Kalfas S; Andersson M; Edwardsson S; Forsgren A; Naidu AS; Human lactoferrin binding to Porphyromonas gingivalis, Prevotella intermedia and Prevotella melaninogenica. Oral Microbiol Immunol 1991 Dec;6(6):350-5.

Kim. K. et ad.: "In Vitro and In Vivo Neutralizing Activity of Human Colostrum and Milk Against Purified Toxins A and B of Clostridium Difficle. J of Infectious Diseases (1984) Vol 150(1) 57-61,

Knutton. Stuart. et ad.: Adhesion of enteropathogenic Escherichia coli to human intestinal enterocytes and cultured human intestinal mucosa. Infection and immunity, Jan 1987. 69-77.

Koenig HL; Schumacher M, Ferraz B. Thi AN: et al: Progesterone synthesis and myedin formation by Schwann cells. Laboratolre Neurobiodogie du Developpement. Unilverslte Bordeaux I, Talence. France. Science 1995 Jun 9:268(5216): 1500-3.

Kohl, S.. et ad: "Human Colostral Cytotoxicity: 1. Antibody Dependent Cellular Cytoxdty Against Herpes Simplex Viral-Infected Cells Mediated by Codostesl Cells" Journal of Clinical Laboratory immuhology (1978) Vol. 1, 221-224.

Korhonen H; Syvaoja EL; et al: Bactericidal effect of bovine normal and immune serum, colostrum and milk against Helicobacter pylori. Valio Research & Development Centre, Helsinki, Finland. J Appl Bacteriol 1995 Jun;78(6):655-62.

Kuwata H; Yip TT; Tomita M; Hutchens TW; Direct evidence of the generation in human stomach of an antimicrobial peptide domain (lactoferricin) from ingested lactoferrin. Department of Food Science and Technology,University of California, Davis Biochi Blophys Acta 1998 Dec8; 1429(1):129-41.

Laine P; Kaartinen M; Penttila A; Panula P; Paavonen T; Kovanen P; Association between myocardial infarction and the mast cells in the adventitia of the infarct-related coronary artery. Wihuri Research Institute, Helsinki, Finland. Circulation 1999 Jan 26;99(3):361-9.

Lacka B; Grzeszczak W; Genetic aspects of diabetic retinopathy. Wiad Lek 1998;51 Suppl 2:24-9.

Lassus, A.; Colosinin Treatment of aphthous ulcers on the oral mucosa. A placedbo-eontmlled study. Dept of Deinniatodogy. U of Helsinid, Finland. International conference of antimicrobic activity of non-antibloties. Copenhagen. Denmark. 1990.

Lee, CS., et ad, "'Local immunity in the mammary gland'" Veterinary Immunology and immunopatlnyodogy, 32 (1992)1-11.

Lee SS: Lawton JW: Chan CE: Li CS: Kwan Th: Chau EF: Antilactofenin antibody in systemic lupus erythematosus. Medical A. Unit. Queen Elizabeth Hospital. Kowloon, Hong Kong. Br J Rheumatol 1992 Oct.31(l0):669-73.

Leszek J; Inglot AD; Janusz M; et al; Colostrinin: a proline-rich polypeptide (PRP) complex isolated from ovine colostrum for treatment of Alzheimer's disease. A double-blind, placebo-controlled study. Psychiatric Unit, Univ. Medical School, Wroclaw, Poland. Arch Immunol Ther Exp (Warsz) 1999;47(6):377-85.

Lindlahr, H. Philosophy of Natural Therapeutics." LindlahrPublishing Co, Chicago, Ill, 1919)

Lin HH: Kao JH: Hsu HY: et al: Absence of infection in breast-fed infants born to hepatitis C virus-infected mothers J Pediatr 1995 Api-, 126(4): 589-91.

Lipsitch M; Bergstrom CT; Levin BR; Department of Biology, Emory University, and Department of Epidemiology, Harvard School of Public Health, Proc Natl Acad Sci U S A 2000 Feb 15;97(4):1938-1943.

Li YM; Glycation ligand binding motif in lactoferrin. Implications in diabetic infection. Adv Exp Med Biol 1998;443:57-63.

Li YM; Tan AX; Vlassara H; Antibacterial activity of lysozyme and lactoferrin is inhibited by binding of advanced glycation-modified proteins to a conserved motif. Nat Med 1995 Oct;1(10):1057-6.

Lissner R; Schmidit H; Karch H; A standard immunoglobulin preparation produced from bovine colostra shows antibody reactivity and neutralization activity against Shiga- like toxins and EHEC-hemolysin of Escherichia coli O157:H7. Biotest Pharma GmbH, Dreieich, Germany. Infection 1996 Sep-Oct;24(5):378-83.

Lonnerdal, B; Iyer, S; Lactoferrin: Molecular Structure and Biological Function, Annu Rev. Nutrition, 1995: 13: 93-110.

Lu M; Yao F; Guo A; A study on two gut hormones in breast milki Research Unit of Pediatrics. Xu zhou Medical College. Chung Hun Pu Cham Ko Tsa Chlh 1995 Oct;30(d0):554-6.

Lu XS: Delfi-alasy JF: Grangeot-Keros L Rannou MT Pllot J Rapid and constant detection of HIV antibody response in saliva of HIV-infected patients; selective distribution of anti-HIV activity in the IgG Isotype. Clamart France. Res Viml 1994 Nov-Dec: 145(61:369-77.

Lupia E; Elliot SJ; Lenz O; Zheng F; Hattori M; Striker GE; Striker LJ; IGF-1 decreases collagen degradation in diabetic NOD mesangial cells: implications for diabetic nephropathy. University of Miami School of Medicine, Florida. Diabetes 1999 Aug;48(8):1638-44.

Machnicki M; Zimecki M; Zagulski T Lactoferrin regulates the release of tumour necrosis factor alpha and interleukin 6 in vivo.   Laboratory of Immunobiology, Polish Academy of Sciences, Wroclaw. Int J Exp Pathol 1993 Oct;74(5):433-9.

Maimone D; Guazzi GC; Annunziata P IL-6 detection in multiple sclerosis brain. Institute of Neurological Sciences, University of Siena, Italy. J Neurol Sci 1997 Feb 27;146(1):59-65.

Majumdar. Anis A et ad "Protective Propertels of Antichodera Antibodies in Human Colostrum," Infection and immunology. Vol 36, No 36. no.3(1982] pp 962-965.

Manev V; Maneva A; Sirakov L; Effect of lactoferrin on the phagocytic activity of polymorphonuclear leuco-cytes isolated from blood of patients with autoimmune diseases and Staphylococcus aureus allergy. Sofia, Bulgaria. Adv Exp Med Biol 1998;443:321-30.

Mann, D; Romm,-E; Migliorini,-M. (1994). Delineation of the glycosaminoglycan-binding site in the human inflammatory response protein lactoferrin. J.Biol.Chem. 269,38: 23661-23667.

Manning, A. "The evolution of infections", USA TODAY, 09-30-1997, pp. 04D.

Marchetti M; Pisani S; Antonini G; Valenti P; Seganti L; Orsi N; Metal complexes of bovine lactoferrin inhibit in vitro replication of herpes simplex virus type 1 and 2. Institute of Microbiology, University of Rome La Sapienza, Italy. Biometals 1998 Apr;11(2):89-94.

Markusse HM: van Haexingen W: Swaak AJ; Hogeweg M; de Jong PT Tear fluid analysis in primary Sjogren's syndrome. Clin Exp Rheumatol. 1993 Mar-Apr,1 1(2T:175-8.

Marone G; de Crescenzo G; et al; Immunological modulation of human cardiac mast cells. Divisione di Immunologia Clinica e Allergologia, Universita di Napoli Federico II, Italy.   Neurochem Res 1999 Sep;24(9):1195-202.

Martinez-Gomis J; Fernandez-Solanas A; et al; Effects of topical application of free and liposome-encapsulat-ed lactoferrin and lactoperoxidase on oral microbiota and dental caries in rats. Arch Oral Biol 1999 Nov;44(11):901-6.

Mattsby-Baltzer I; Roseanu A; Motas C; Elverfors J; et al; Lactoferrin or a fragment thereof inhibits the endo-toxin-induced interleukin-6 response in human monocytic cells. Department of Clinical Bacteriology, University of Goteborg, Sweden. Pediatr Res 1996 Aug;40(2):257-62.

Matsuda, T. et al; Il-6/BSF2 in Normal and Abnormal Regultion of Immune Responses, Annals of the New York Academy of Sciences, 1989, Vol: 557, NYAS, NY, 466-476.

McClane SJ; Rombeau JLCytokines and inflammatory bowel disease: a review. Hospital of the University of Pennsylvania, Philadelphia JPEN J Parenter Enteral Nutr 1999 Sep-Oct;23(5 Suppl):S20-4.

Mero A; Miikkulainen H; Riski J; Pakkanen R; Aalto J; Takala T; Effects of bovine colostrum supplementation on serum IGF-I, IgG, hormone, and saliva IgA during training. University of Jyvaskyla, 40351 Jyvaskyla, Finland. J Appl Physiol 1997 Oct;83(4):1144-51.

Miyauchi H; Hashimoto S; Nakajima M; et al; Bovine lactoferrin stimulates the phagocytic activity of human neutrophils: identification of its active domain.Japan.Cell Immunol 1998 Jul 10;187(1):34-7.

Moddoveanu, Zina, et al: Antibacterial Properties of Milk: IgA Peroxidase-Lactoferrir Interactions. Annals of N.Y. Academy of Science (1983) Vol 409.848-850.

Moldofsky H; Sleep, neuroimmune and neuroendocrine functions in fibromyalgia and chronic fatigue syn-drome. Adv Neuroimmunol 1995;5(1):39-56.

Molnar I, et al.; High circulating IL-6 level in Graves' ophthalmopathy. Autoimmunity. 1997;25(2):91-6.

Moniuszko T; Rutkowski R; Chyrek-Borowska S; Production of selected cytokines by monocytes (IL-1 beta, IL-6) and lymphocytes (IL-2, IL-4) in peripheral blood of patients with nonallergic bronchial asthma treated with Broncho-Vaxom. Pneumonol Alergol Pol 1995;63 Suppl 2:66-70.

Murphey DK; Buescher ES: Human colosirum has anti-inflammatory activity in a rat subcutaneous ar pouch model of inflammatton. Pedlatr Res 1993 Aiig:34(2):208-12. Newberne. P.M.. Young. V.R, Nature (March 23. 1973).

Nakao K; Imoto I; Ikemura N; Shibata T; et al; Relation of lactoferrin levels in gastric mucosa with Helicobacter pylori infection and with the degree of gastric inflammation. Am J Gastroenterol 1997 Jun;92 (6):1005-11.

Nakao K; Imoto I; Gabazza EC; Yamauchi K; et al; Gastric juice levels of lactoferrin and Helicobacter pylori infection. Scand J Gastroenterol 1997 Jun;32(6):530-4.

Naudin J; Mege JL; Azorin JM; Dassa D; Elevated circulating levels of IL-6 in schizophrenia. Service du Pr Azorin, CHU Sainte-Marguerite, Marseille, France. Schizophr Res 1996 Jul 5;20(3):269-73.

Nawata, Y., et al; Il-6 is the Principal Factor Produced by Synovia of Patients with Rheumatoid Arthritis that induces B-lymphocytes to secrete immunoglobulins. Annals of the New York Academy of Sciences, 1989, Vol: 557, NYAS, NY, 230-238.

Neurath MF; Fuss I; Schurmann G; Pettersson S; Arnold K; Muller-Lobeck H; Strober W; Herfarth C; Buschenfelde KHCytokine gene transcription by NF-kappa B family members in patients with inflammatory bowel disease. Laboratory of Immunology, University of Mainz, Germany. Ann N Y Acad Sci 1998 Nov 17;859:149-59.

Neuringer, M.; Reisbick, S.; Janowsky, J.; The Role of n-3 fatty acids is visual and cognitive development: Current edidence and methods of assessment. The Journal of Pediatrics, 1994, Vol. 125,:5, Part 2 S39-S47.

The New England Journal of Medicine, Intravenous Immune Globulln For the Prevention of Bacterial Infections in Children wtth Symptomatic Human Immuno Deficiency Virus Infections.(July 11, 1991)325:73-80.

Noda. Kovichi, et al. Transforming Growth Factor Activity in Human Colostrum: Gannoo (1984) Vol.75, 109-112.

Noni, Jill, Pearl Map David DlJohn, Saul Tsiporoo and Carol O. Tacket: Treatment With Bovine Hyperimmune Colostrum of Cxytosprbdlal Dlanhea in AIDS Patients. AIDS (1990)4:581-584.

Nord J; Ma P; DiJohn D; Tzipori S; Tacket CO; Treatment with bovine hyperimmune colostrum of cryp-tosporidial diarrhea in AIDS patients. St Vincent's Hospital and Medical Center, NY. AIDS 1990 Jun;4(6):581-4.

Ogra. Pearav. et al.: Annals of New York Acedemy of Science. (1983) Vol. 409.82-92.

Ogra. Pearay. et al.; Colosirum derived Immunity and Maternal Neonatal Interaction. Annals of NY Acedemy of Science (1983) Vol. 409, pp 82-92.

Oldham, G.: Suppression of bovine lymphocyte responses to mitogens following in vivo and in vitro treatment with dexamethasone. Veterinary Immunology and Immunophysology, 320 (1992)161-177.

Peen E; Johansson A; Engquist M; Skogh T; Hepatic and extrahepatic clearance of circulating human lacto-ferrin: an experimental study in rat. Department of Medical Microbiology, Faculty of Health Sciences,

Linkoping University, Sweden. Eur J Haematol 1998 Sep;61(3):151-9.

Pell, J.M.. and Bates, P.C.; Manipulation of growth and muscle protein metabolism by exogenous insulin-like growth-factor 1 and growth hormone. Acts Paedlair Scand (Supple) 367:161.

Petschow BW; Talbott RD; Batema RP; Ability of lactoferrin to promote the growth of Bifidobacterium spp.in vitro is independent of receptor binding capacity and iron saturation level. J Med Microbio l1999 Jun;48(6):541-9.

Plettenberg A Stoehr A Stellbrink I-U; Albrecht H MeigelW.: A preparation from bovine colostrun in the treatment of HIV-positive patients with chronic diarrhea. Clin Investig 1993 Jam7l(1):42-5.

Pollanen MT; Hakkinen L; Overman DO; Salonen JI; Lactoferrin impedes epithelial cell adhesion in vitro. J Periodontal Res 1998 Jan;33(1):8-16

Prokopiv MM: Iarosh AA. Effect of colostnim on the enzymatic function of the liver in patients with multiple sclerosisi. Vrach Delo 1988 Apr,(4): 100-2.

Puddu P; Borghi P; Gessani S; et al; Antiviral effect of bovine lactoferrin saturated with metalions on early steps of human immunodeficiency virus type1 infection. Int J Biochem Cell Biol 1998 Sep 30(9):1055-62.

Punzi L, et al. Interrelationship between synovial fluid interleukin (IL)-6, IL-1 beta and disease activity indices in rheumatoid arthritis. Rheumatol Int. 1994;14(2):83-4.

Rice KD; Tanaka RD; Katz BA; Numerof RP; Moore WRInhibitors of tryptase for the treatment of mast cell-mediated diseases. Curr Pharm Des 1998 Oct;4(5):381-96.

Rodriguez-Ortega. Morella. et al.; Membrane glycoproteins of humm polymorphonuclear leukocytes that act as receptors for mannose-specific escherichia coli. Infection and Immunity. April 1987, 968-973.

Rodriguez M; Pavelko KD; McKinney CW; Leibowitz JL Recombinant human IL-6 suppresses demyelination in a viral model of multiple sclerosis. Department of Neurology, Mayo Clinic, Rochester, MN. J Immunol 1994 Oct 15;153(8):3811-21.

Rogler G; Meinel A; Lingauer A; Michl J; Zietz B; Gross V; Lang B; Andus T; Scholmerich J; Palitzsch KD; Glucocorticoid receptors are down-regulated in inflamed colonic mucosa but not in peripheral blood mononuclear cells from patients with inflammatory bowel disease. Eur J Clin Invest 1999 Apr;29(4):330-6.

Rouse. B.T., et al.: Antibody-Dependent Cell Mediated Cytotoxicity in Cows: Comparison of Effector Cell Activity Against Heterologous Erythrocyte and Herpes virus-infected Bovine Target Cells. Infection and immunity (1976) Vol 13. 1433.

Rump JA Arndt K Arnold A Bendick C: Diehteimuller H: Franke M; Heim EB: Jager H: Kampmann B: Kolb P: et ad.: Treatment of diarrhea in human immunodeficiency virus-infected patients with immunoglobulins from bovine codostrum. Clin Investig 1992 Jul;70(71:588-94.

Saha K Dun N: Chopra K Use of human colostrum in the management of chronic infantile diarrhea due to enteropathogenic E. coli infection with associated intestinal parasite infestations and undernutrition. J TropPediair 1990 Oct:36(51 :247-50.

Saito H; Asakura K; Ogasawara H; et al; Topical antigen provocation increases the number of immunoreactive IL-4- , IL-5- and IL-6-positive cells in the nasal mucosa of patients with perennial allergic rhinitis. Int Arch Allergy Immunol 1997 Sep;114(1):81-5.

Sallh, Y.. LR McDowell, J.F. Hentges. R.M. Mason. C.J. Wilcox: Mineral Content of Milk, Colostrum, and Serum as Affected by Physiological State and Mineral Supplementation. Journal of Dairy Science (1987) Vol.70(5), 608-612.

Samborski W; Lacki JK; Wiktorowicz KE; The lymphocyte phenotype in patients with primary fibromyalgia. Ups J Med Sci 1996;101(3):251-6.

Samnson. R., et al.: Inununology (1979) Vol. 381 (2), 376-73.

Saniholm. M.. et ad, (1979) Colostral Trypsin-Inhibitor Capacity in Different Animal Species, Acta Veteninaria Scandinavica. Vol. 20. (41.469-476.

Sarker SA; Casswall TH; Mahalanabis D;et al; Successful treatment of rotavirus diarrhea in children with immunoglobulin from immunized bovine colostrum. Pediatr Infect Dis J 1998 Dec;17(12):1149-54.

Schmidt AM, et al. Regulation of human mononuclear phagocyte migration by cell surface-binding proteins for advanced glycation end products. J Clin Invest. 1993 May;91(5):2155-68.

Segev Y; Landau D; et al; Growth hormone receptor antagonism prevents early renal changes in nonobese diabetic mice. J Am Soc Nephrol 1999 Nov;10(11):2374-81.

Shing. Yuen and Elagabrun, Micheal: Purification and characterization of a bovine Colostrumderived growth factor. Molecular Endocrinolocy 1987, 335.

Siciliano R, et al. Bovine lactoferrin peptidic fragments involved in inhibition of herpes simplex virus type 1 infection. Biochem Biophys Res Commun. 1999 Oct 14;264(1):19-23.

Singleton, P; Sainsbury, D.; Dictionary of Microbiology and Molecular Biology, 2nd ed. 1996. Wiley.

Skotiner, V.: Anabolic and Tilsue Repair Functions of Recombinant Insulin-Like Growth Factors I, Acta Pediatr Scand (Suppll 376:367:63-66, 1990.

Snydennan. Ralph, M.D.: Advances in Rheumatology. Medical Clinics of North America. (Mamth 1986) Vol.70(21,217.

Sporn, MB.. et al. "Polypeptide Transforming Growth Factors Isolated From Bovine Sources and used for Wound Healing in Vivo" Science (1983) Vol 219. 1329-1331.

Staroscik, K., et al. "Immunologically Active Nonapeptide Fragment of a Proline-Rich Polypeptide from Ovine-Colostrum: Amino And Sequence and Immuno-regulatoiy Properties" Molecular immunology (1983) Vol. 20(121. 1277-1282.

Stromqvist M; Falk P; Bergstrom S; Hansson L; et al; Human milk kappa-casein and inhibition of Helicobacter pylori adhesion to human gastric mucosa. J Pediatr Gastroenterol Nutr 1995 Oct;21(3):288-96.

Subratty AH; Hooloman NK; Role of circulating inflammatory cytokines in patients during an acute attack of bronchial asthma.   Indian J Chest Dis Allied Sci 1998 Jan-Mar;40(1):17-21.

Swaak AJ, et al. Cytokine production (IL-6 and TNF alpha) in whole blood cell cultures ofpatients with systemic lupus erythematosus. Scand J Rheumatol. 1996;25(4):233-8.

Ritchie, and Becker 1994 titis Update on the management of intestinal cryptosporidlosis in AIDS. Ann-Pharmacol. 28:767-78

Rouse. B.T. et at.. 1976. Antibodydependent Cell-mediated cytotoxicity in cows: Comparison of cifector cell activity against heterologous erythroeytes and herpesrus-infected bovine target cells. Infect. Immun. 13:1 433A0.

Salvi M, et al. Increased serum concentrations of interleukin-6 (IL-6) and soluble IL-6 receptor in patients with Graves' disease. J Clin Endocrinol Metab. 1996 Aug;81(8):2976-9.

Swart PJ: Kulpers ME: et al; Antiviral effects of milk pmteins: acylation results in polyanionic compounds with potent activity against human immunodeficiency virus types I and 2 in vitro. AIDS Res Hum Retroviruses 1996 Jun 10: 12(9):769-75

Swart PJ: Kulpers ME: et al.: Antiviral effects of milk proteins: acylation results in polyanionic compounds with potent activity against human immunodeficiency virus types I and 2 in vitro. AIDS Res Hum Reimviruses 1996 Jun 10: 12(9):769-75.

Swart, P.J et al. (1996). Antiviral effects of milk proteins: Acylation results in polyanionic compounds with potent activity against human immunodeficiency virus types I and 2 in vitro. AIDS-RES-HUM-RETROVIRUS-ES. 12,9: 769-775.

Swart PJ; Kuipers EM; Smit C; Van Der Strate BW; Harmsen MC; Meijer DK; Lactoferrin. Antiviral activity of lactoferrin. Department of Pharmacology, University of Groningen, The Netherlands. Adv Exp Med Biol 1998;443:205-13.

Tanaka K; Ikeda M; Nozaki A; Kato N; Tsuda H; Saito S; Sekihara H. Lactoferrin inhibits hepatitis C virus viremia in patients with chronic hepatitis C: a pilot study. Third Department of Internal Medicine, Yokohama City University School of Medicine, Yokohama. Jpn J Cancer Res 1999 Apr; 90(4):367-71.

Taylor, B, Wadsorth, J; Breastfeeding and child development at five years Developmental Medicine and Child Neurology, 1984, 26. pg. 73-80.

Tenovuo J; Lumikari M; Soukka T; Salivary lysozyme, lactoferrin and peroxidases: antibacterial effects on cariogenic bacteria and clinical applications in preventive dentistry. Proc Finn Dent Soc 1991;87(2):197-208.

Theodore, Christine. et al.; "Immunologic Aspects of Colostrum and Milk: Development of Antibody Response to Respiratory Syncytial Virus and Bovine Serum Albumin in the Human and Rabbit Mammary Gland" Recent Advances in Mucosal Immunity (1982) (Raven Preas), New York.

Tokuyama H: Tokuyama Y: Bovine colostre transforming growth factor-beta-like peptide that induces growth inhibition and changes in morphology of human osteogenic sarcoma cells (MG63). Cell Biol int Rep 1989 Mar.13(3):251-8.

Thomas, Frank et al.: Increased weight gain, nitrogen retention and muscle protein zynthesis following treatment of dinbetic rats with IGF-I anddes 1-3 (IGF-II. BlochemJ. 1991,276: 547- 554- 547

Thomas. Frank et a.; Effects of full-length and trunicated insulin-like growth factor-l on nitrogen balance and muscle protein metaholism in nitrogen restrcted rate. J Endocrinology 1991, 128: 97-105.

Toner, M. "Science Watch: Antibiotics' Nemesis: Bacteria that become resistant to the 20th century's wonder drugs are: hardier, longer-lasting adversaries than scientists had suspected." The Atlanta Journal and Constitution; 12-07-1997.

Tritschler, P. HJ, Wolff, S.P., Thioctic (lipoic) acid: a therapeutic metal-chelating antioxidant? Biochem Pharmacol 1995 Jun 29;50(1):123-6.

Tsai WJ: Uu HW: Yen JH: Chen JR Lin SF: Chen TP: Lactoferrin in rheumatoid arthritis and systemic lupus erythematous. Kao Hsiung I Hsueh Ku Hsueh Tsa Chili 1991 Jan: 7(l):22-6.

Tzipori 5: Roberton D; Cooper DA: White L; Chronic cryptosporidlal diarrhea and hyperimmune cow colostrum Idetterd. Lancet 1987 Aug 8:2(8554):344-5.

Tyrell, David.: Breast Feeding and Virus Infection The Immunity of Infant Feeding. (1980) Plenum Press, N.Y.. 55-61.

Ulcova-Gallova Z, et al.; Immunologic factors in human colostrum and milk. Cas Lek Cesk. 1994 May 2;133(9):275-6.

Urban, T. The Oponizing ability in antibodies from some health care products containing bovine colostrum. State Laboratory, State Pharmaceutical Company. Stockholm. Swedish Pharmaceutical Asociation, Yearly Congress, 1990.

van Leeuwen MA; Westra J; Limburg PC; van Riel PL; van Rijswijk MH Interleukin-6 in relation to other proinflammatory cytokines, chemotactic activity and neutrophil activation in rheumatoid synovial fluid. Ann Rheum Dis 1995 Jan;54(1):33-8.

Vassilev it: Veleva KV: Natoral polyreactive IgA and IgM autoantibodies in human colosinim. Seand J immunol 1996 Nov.44(5):535-9.

Viander B: Ala-Uotila 5: Jalkanen NI: Pakkanen R, Viable AC-2. a new adult bovine serum- and codostrum-based supplement for the culture of mammalian cells. Blotechniques 1996 Apr,20(41:702-7.

Von Fellenberg, Fl.; Hoeber, H;: Multiple protease Inhibitors in and Codosinim and in bovine udder tissue and their possible significance. Schwelz. Arch. Tierheilkd. 1980.122 (31. 159-66.

Vorland LH; Ulvatne H; Andersen J; Haukland H; Rekdal O;et al; Lactoferricin of bovine origin is more active than lactoferricins of human, murine and caprine origin. Scand J Infect Dis 1998;30(5):513-7.

Wada T; Aiba Y; Shimizu K; Takagi A; Miwa T; Koga Y; The therapeutic effect of bovine lactoferrin in the host infected with Helicobacter pylori. Scand J Gastroenterol 1999 Mar;34(3):238-43.

Wads. N. et al.: Neutralizing Activity Against Clxxstridium Difficile Toxins in the Supernatant of Cultured Colostral Cells. Inictious Immunology (1980) Vol 29.545-550.

Ward, C.G. Bullen, J.J., Rogers, H.J.; Iron and Infection: New Developments and their Implications, Journ of Trauma, Injury, Infection and Critical Care, 1996, Vol 41:2, 356-364.

Wadsteinm J, The use of colosirum immuglobulines against gastrointestinal disorders, mouth infections and cutaneous infections, University of Lond. Sweden (Feb 1991).

Wakabayashi H; Okutomi T; Abe S; Hayasawa H; Tomita M; Yamaguchi Hy, Morinaga Enhanced anti-Candida activity of neutrophils and azole antifungal agents in the presence of lactoferrin-related compounds. Adv Exp Med Bio l1998;443:229-37.

Ward, P.P; Zhou, X; Conneely, O.M. (1996). Cooperative interactions between the amino-and carboxyl- terminal lobes contribute to the unique iron-binding stability of lactoferrin. J. Biol. Chem. 271,22: 12790-12794.

Watanabe T; Nagura H; Watanabe K; et al The binding of human milk lactoferrin to immunoglobulin A. FEBS Left 1984 Mar 26: 168(2):203-7.

Weldham, RH., et al; Annals of N.Y. Academy of Science., (1983) 409. 510-515.

Welle MM; Olivry T; Grimm S; Suter M; Mast cell density and subtypes in the skin of dogs with atopic dermatitis. J Comp Pathol 1999 Feb;120(2):187-97.

Wester TJ; Fiorotto ML; Klindt J; Burrin DG; Feeding colostrum increases circulating insulin-like growth factor I in newborn pigs independent of endogenous growth hormone secretion. ARS, USDA, Department of Pediatrics, Baylor College of Medicine, Houston, TX. J Anim Sci 1998 Dec;76(12):3003-9.

Wlaszczyk A; Zimecki M; Adamik B; Durek G; Kubler A: Immunological status of patients subjected to cardiac surgery: effect of lactoferrin on proliferation and production of interleukin 6 and tumor necrosis factor alpha by peripheral blood mononuclear cells in vitro. Arch Immunol Ther Exp (Warsz) 1997;45(2-3):201-12.

Wootan, George, "Take Charge of Your Child's Health"" Crown Publishers. Inc. New York (1992) pg 111-135.

Wong WW: Hachey DL: Insull W: Opekun AR, Klein PD: Effect of dietary cholesterol on cholesterol synthesis in breast-fed and formula-fed infants. USDA/ARS Children's Nutrition Research Center, Department of Pediatrics, Baylor College of Medicine, Houston, TX. J Lipid Flea 1993 Aug:34(81:1403-11.

Woywodt A; Ludwig D; et al: Mucosal cytokine expression, cellular markers and adhesion molecules in inflammatory bowel disease. Eur J Gastroenterol Hepatol 1999 Mar;11(3):267-76.

Xu Ri: Development of the newborn Gl tract and is relation to codostrum/milk intake: a review. Department of Zoology, University of Hong Kong, Reprod Fertil Dev 1996:8(11:35-48.

XuY Y; Samaranayake YH; Samaranayake LP; Nikawa H Invitro susceptibility of Candida species to lactoferrin. School of Stomatology, Beijing Medical University, China. Med Mycol 1999 Feb; 37(1):35-41.

Yamauchi K; Wakabayashi H; Hashimoto S; Teraguchi S Hayasawa H; Tomita M.; Effects of orally administered bovine lactoferrin on the immune system of healthy volunteers. Adv Exp Med Biol 1998;443:261-5.

Yavuzyilmaz E; Yumak O; Akdoganli T; et al; The alterations of whole saliva constituents in patients with diabetes mellitus. Aust Dent J 1996 Jun;41(3):193-7.

Ye S: Sun R, Lu 9: The study of growth factors in human colostrmm. Nanjing University.

Yoo YC; Watanabe S; Watanabe R; Hata K; Shimazaki K; et al., Bovine lactoferrin and Lactoferricin inhibit tumor metastasis in mice. Adv Exp Med Biol 1998;443:285-91.

Zimecki M; Spiegel K; Wlaszczyk A; Kubler A; Kruzel ML; Lactoferrin increases the output of neutrophil precursors and attenuates the spontaneous production of TNF-alpha and IL-6 by peripheral blood cells..Arch Immunol Ther Exp (Warsz) 1999;47(2):113-8.

Zimecki M; Wlaszczyk A; Cheneau P; Brunel A; et al; Immunoregulatory effects of a nutritional preparation containing bovine lactoferrin taken orally by healthy individuals. Institute of Immunology and Experimental Therapy, Polish Academy of Sciences, Wroclaw, Poland. Arch Immunol Ther Exp (Warsz) 1998;46(4):231-40.

Zimecki M; Miedzybrodzki R; Szymaniec S Oral treatment of rats with bovine lactoferrin inhibits carrageenan-induced inflammation; correlation with decreased cytokine production. Arch Immunol Ther Exp (Warsz) 1998;46(5):361-5.

Zimecki M; Wlaszczyk A Zagulski T; Kubler A; Lactoferrin lowers serum interleukin 6 and tumor necrosis factor alpha levels in mice subjected to surgery. Arch Immunol Ther Exp (Warsz) 1998;46(2):97-104.

INDEX

ABOUT THE AUTHOR

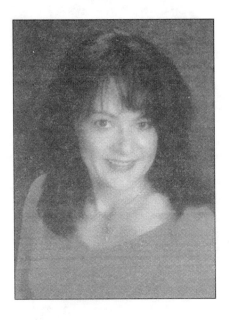

Beth M. Ley, Ph.D., has been a science writer specializing in health and nutrition for over 10 years and has written over a dozen health related books, including the best sellers, **DHEA: Unlocking the Secrets to the Fountain of Youth** and **MSM: On Our Way Back to Health With Sulfur**. She wrote her own undergraduate degree program and graduated in Scientific and Technical Writing from North Dakota State University in 1987 (combination of Zoology and Journalism). Beth has her masters (1997) and doctoral degrees (1999) in Nutrition.

Beth lives in the Minnesota lakes country. She is dedicated to God and to spreading the health message. She enjoys spending time with her Dalmatians, exercises on a regular basis, eats a vegetarian, low-fat diet and takes anti-aging supplements.

Memberships: American Academy of Anti-aging, New York Academy of Sciences, Oxygen Society.

YOU NEED TO KNOW...
THE HEALTH MESSAGE

Do you not know that you are God's temple and that God's Spirit dwells in you? If anyone destroys God's temple, God will destroy him, For God's temple is holy and that temple you are.
1 Corinthians 3:16-17

So, whether you eat or drink, or whatever you do, do all to the glory of God.
1 Corinthians 10:31

ORDER THESE GREAT BOOKS
FROM BL PUBLICATIONS!

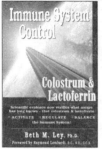

Immune System Control
Colostrum & Lactoferrin
Beth M. Ley, Ph.D. 200 pages, $12.95 ISBN 1-890766-11-9
Get the indepth and detailed FACTS about colostum and lactoferrin! Testimonials and much more! Also features a special product selection guide! Fully referenced/Indexed

Marvelous Memory Boosters
Beth M. Ley, Ph.D. 2000, 32 pages, $3.95

Certain nutrients & phytochemicals (Alpha GPC, Vinpocetine, Huperzine-A, Pregnenolone, Phospholipids, DHA, Bacopa Monniera, Ginkgo Biloba, etc.) improve short & long term memory, increase mental acuity & concentration, improve learning abilities & mental stamina, reduce fatigue, improve sleep, mood, vision & hearing.

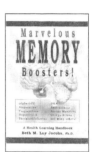

Aspirin Alternatives:
The Top Natural Pain-Relieving Analgesics
Raymond Lombardi, D.C., N.D., C.C.N., 1999, 160 pages, $8.95

This book discusses analgesics and natural approaches to pain. Ibuprofen and acetaminophen are used for pain-relief, but like all drugs, there is a risk of side effects and interactions, There are a number of natural alternatives which are equally effective and in many cases may be preferable because they may help treat the underlining problem rather than simply treating a symptom.

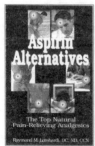

Vinpocetine: Boost Your Brain w/ Periwinkle
Extract! Beth M. Ley, Ph.D. 2000, 48 pgs. $4.95

This herbal extract benefits: Memory, attention and concentration, learning, circulation, hearing, insomnia, depression, tinnitus, vision & more! Vinpocetine increases circulation in the brain and increases metabolism in the brain by increasing use of glucose and oxygen. Benefits both the old and young!

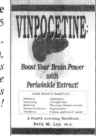

Coenzyme Q10: All Around
Nutrient for All-Around Health!
Beth M. Ley-Jacobs, Ph.D., 1999, 60 pages, $4.95

CoQ10 is found in every living cell. With age, insufficient levels become more common, putting us at serious risk of illness and disease. Protect and strengthen the cardiovascular system; benefit blood pressure, immunity, fatigue, weight problems, Alzheimer's, Parkinson's, Huntington's, gum-disease and slow aging.

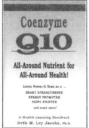

78

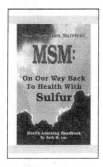

MSM: On Our Way Back To Health With Sulfur Beth M. Ley, 1998, 40 pages, $3.95

MSM (methyl sulfonyl methane), is a rich source of organic sulfur, important for connective tissue regeneration. Beneficial for arthritis and other joint problems, allergies, asthma, skin problems, TMJ, periodontal conditions, pain relief, and much more! Includes important "How to use" directions.

How to Fight Osteoporosis & Win: The Miracle of MCHC
Beth M. Ley, 80 pgs. $6.95

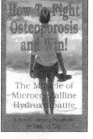

Find out if you are at risk for osteroporosis and what to do to prevent and reverse it. Get the truth about bone loss, calcium, supplements, foods, MCHC & much more! Find out what supplements can help you most!

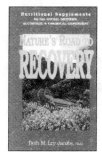

Nature's Road to Recovery: Nutritional Supplements for The Social Drinker, Alcoholic & Chemical-Dependent
Beth M. Ley-Jacobs, Ph.D., 1999, 72 pages, $5.95

Recovery involves much more than abstinence. Cravings, depression, memory loss, liver problems, vascular problems, sexual problems, sleep problems, nutritional deficiencies and common health problems which can benefit from 5-HTP, DHA, phospholipids, St. John's Wort, antioxidants, etc.

DHA: The Magnificent Marine Oil
Beth M. Ley-Jacobs, Ph.D., 1999, 120 pages, $6.95

Individuals commonly lack this essential Omega-3 fatty acid so important to the brain, vision, and immune system and much more. Memory, depression, ADD, addiction disorders (especially alcoholism), inflammatory disorders, skin problems, schizophrenia, elevated blood lipids, etc., benefit from DHA.

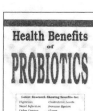

Health Benefits of Probiotics
Dr. S.K. Dash & Dr. Allen Spreen 2000, 56 pages, $4.95

Probiotics aid in the maintenance of the healthy balance of intestinal flora. They improve digestion, cholesterol levels, immunity; Correct digestive disorders, ulcers, inflammatory bowel diseases, lactose intolerance, yeast infections; Help prevent colon cancer; Reduce side effects of antibiotics & more!

Look for these titles from BL PUBLICATIONS in your local health food or book stores or

TO   PLACE   AN   ORDER:

# of copies

_____ *Aspirin Alternatives: The Top Natural Pain-Relieving Analgesics* (Lombardi) $8.95

_____ *Castor Oil: Its Healing Properties* (Ley) $3.95

_____ *Dr. John Willard on Catalyst Altered Water* (Ley) $3.95

_____ *Coenzyme Q10: All-Around Nutrient for All-Around Health* (Ley Jacobs) $4.95

_____ *Colostrum: Nature's Gift to the Immune System* (Ley) . $5.95

_____ *DHA: The Magnificent Marine Oil* (Ley Jacobs) $6.95

_____ *DHEA: Unlocking the Secrets of the Fountain of Youth- 2nd Edition* (Ash- Ley) $14.95

_____ *Health Benefits of Probiotics* (Dash) $4.95

_____ *How Did We Get So Fat?* (Susser) $7.95

_____ *How to Fight Osteoporosis and Win! The Miracle of Microcrystalline Hydroxyapatite* (Ley) $6.95

_____ *Immune System Control- Colostrum & Lactoferrin* (Ley) $12.95

_____ *Marvelous Memory Boosters* (Ley) $3.95

_____ *MSM: On Our Way Back to Health W/ Sulfur* (Ley) ... $3.95

_____ *Natural Healing Handbook* (Ley) $14.95

_____ *Nature's Road to Recovery: Nutritional Supplements for the Alcoholic & Chemical Dependent* (Ley Jacobs) $5.95

_____ *PhytoNutrients: Medicinal Nutrients Found in Foods* (Ley) $3.95

_____ *The Potato Antioxidant: Alpha Lipoic Acid* (Ley) $6.95

_____ *Vinpocetine: Revitalize Your Brain with Periwinkle Extract!* (Ley) $4.95

Book subtotal $ _____   Please add $3.00 for shipping

TOTAL $_____

Send check or money order to:
BL Publications 14325 Barnes Drive Detroit Lakes, MN 56501

Credit card orders call toll free: 1-877-BOOKS11

Orders may also be placed online at: www.supplementshopper.com